Sunset

diabetic
cookbook

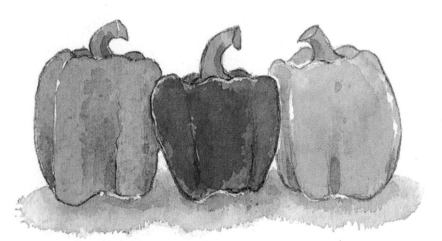

By the Editors of Sunset Books

Sunset Publishing Corporation Menlo Park, CA

SUNSET BOOKS

President & Publisher: Susan J. Maruyama

Director, Sales & Marketing: Richard A. Smeby

Editorial Director: Bob Doyle

Production Director: Lory Day

Art Director: Vasken Guiragossian

Retail Sales Development Manager: Becky Ellis

SUNSET PUBLISHING CORPORATION

Chairman: Jim Nelson

President/Chief Executive Officer: Stephen J. Seabolt

Chief Financial Officer: James E. Mitchell

Publisher: Anthony P. Glaves

Director of Finance: Larry Diamond

Vice President, Manufacturing: Lorinda B. Reichert

Editor, Sunset Magazine: Rosalie Muller Wright

Senior Editor, Food & Entertaining: Jerry Anne Di Vecchio

The *Sunset Diabetic Cookbook* was produced in conjunction with Rebus, Inc., New York, NY.

Editor and Publisher: Rodney M. Friedman

Associate Publisher: Barbara Maxwell O'Neill

Editor in Chief: Charles L. Mee, Jr.

Staff for this Book

Executive Editor: Marya Dalrymple

Developmental Editor: Linda J. Selden

Design: Karin Martin

Illustrations: Mary Haverfield

Editorial Assistant: Rebecca Porter

Dietary Consultant: Patricia Kearney, R.D., Stanford University Hosptial

Nutritional Analysis: Hill Nutrition Associates, Inc.

Production Coordinator: Patricia S. Williams

ABOUT THIS BOOK

The *Sunset Diabetic Cookbook* provides healthful delicious food choices for people with or without diabetes. Seven chapters offer recipes for soups, main-course salads, meats, poultry, seafood, meatless entrées, and side dishes—more than 85 choices in all. Though the book doesn't include desserts, that does not mean that desserts are off limits for people with diabetes. To end any meal on a sweet note, try fruit—a ripe peach or pear, a crisp apple, or a bowl of berries is a perfect choice for any occasion.

All of the recipes in this book were developed in the Sunset test kitchens. Each recipe offers a list of Food Exchanges for Meal Planning for diabetics as well as a nutrient analysis (see the Introduction, pages 4–8, for a more detailed explanation), and there are preparation and cooking times given, too. Keep in mind that these times are approximate and will vary depending on your expertise in the kitchen and on the cooking equipment you use.

Whatever your particular needs may be, the *Sunset Diabetic Cookbook* has the solution. Apply these recipes to your nutrition and exercise prescription—and you'll be assured of meeting the guidelines for healthy eating and satisfying your goals for maintaining normal levels of blood glucose and blood lipids.

If you have comments or suggestions, please let us hear from you. Write to us at:

Sunset Books/Cookbook Editorial
80 Willow Road
Menlo Park, CA 94025

To order additional copies of any of our books, call us at 1 (800) 634-3095 or check with your local bookstore.

Front Cover:
Arroz con Pollo (recipe, page 62). Photography by *Chris Shorten;* food styling by *Susan Massey.*

Photography Credits:
Pages 11, 21, 35, 39, 45, 59, 71, 79, 93: photography by *Keith Ovregaard;* photo styling by *Susan Massey;* food styling by *Cynthia Scheer.* Pages 29, 49: photography by *Nikolay Zurek;* photo styling by *Susan Massey.* Pages 65, 103: photography by *Kevin Sanchez;* photo styling by *Susan Massey.* Pages 83, 109: photography by *Allan Rosenberg;* associate photographer, *Allen V. Lott;* photo styling by *Sandra Griswold;* food styling by *Heidi Gintner;* assistant food and photo styling by *Elizabeth C. Davis.* Page 87: photography by *Tom Wyatt;* food styling by *Susan Massey.*

❖ Contents ❖

❖ Introduction ❖

DIABETES & DIET: AN OVERVIEW

Dietary management for people with diabetes mellitus is designed to meet individual blood glucose (sugar) and blood lipid (fat) goals—that is, to keep blood glucose and blood lipid levels as normal as possible. At the same time, the diet you choose must satisfy your calorie requirements for a reasonable body weight and also meet the nutrient needs appropriate to your stage in life. Diabetes can occur at any time from infancy to old age, and each stage has distinct calorie and nutrient demands. Children who have diabetes, for example, need a high-calorie, high-nutrient diet to fuel growth and development, while older women must get enough calcium and vitamin D in order to protect their bones. Meeting these needs, in concert with maintaining optimal blood glucose and blood lipid levels, may stop or slow the progression of diabetes complications involving the eyes, nerves, kidneys, and blood vessels.

Daily food choices, meal patterns, exercise, medication, and self-monitoring of blood glucose are all important in the nutrition and medical management of people with diabetes. Keep in mind that, to meet your diabetes goals and lifestyle needs, you must play an active role in your overall care. Working together, you and your physician, nurse, and dietitian can assess your nutritional and medical status, then set individual treatment goals and identify any need for additional training in diabetes self-management.

DIABETIC FOODS ARE OUT!

Good news—people with diabetes do not have to buy special foods! The recipes in the *Sunset Diabetic Cookbook* are for those interested in healthful eating, whether or not they have diabetes. To help you design your daily menus, each recipe provides a list of Food Exchanges, developed by the American Diabetes Association and the American Dietetic Association, and a nutrient analysis. For optimal control of the nutrients and calories in any dish, be precise about measuring or weighing ingredients; carefully prepared recipes used in your meal plan may improve blood glucose and blood lipid levels. In this book, the ingredient lists and instructions in each recipe give both United States standard measures and metric equivalents for weight, volume, and dimension: 1 tablespoon (15 ml) salad oil, 8 ounces (230 g) mushrooms, a 10- by 15-inch (25- by 38-cm) baking pan, and so on.

EXCHANGE LISTS FOR MEAL PLANNING

The chart on page 6 represents an overview of the Exchange Lists for Meal Planning, a system that helps people with diabetes monitor calorie and nutrient intake, an important aspect of diabetes self-management. The Exchange Lists for Meal Planning groups together foods with a similar amount of carbohydrate, protein, and fat per serving. There are three major groups: carbohydrate, meat and meat substitutes, and fat. Each group is broken down into lists of foods; the carbohydrate group, for example, includes—among others—starch, fruit, and milk lists. If you would like a complete listing of the individual foods in each Exchange List, ordering information can be found at the bottom of the chart. In the complete listing, for each food *within* each list, serving size is specified to provide a particular amount of nutrients and calories per portion. By using the Exchange Lists, you are able to have flexibility in food choices, since any food on a list can be "exchanged," or traded, for any other food on the same list. Every recipe in this book provides the number of Exchanges per serving. Pay close attention to serving size and remember to measure cooked foods as often as possible, just as you should measure each ingredient as you prepare the recipes.

In the *carbohydrate group*, servings from the starch, fruit, and milk lists have a similar carbohydrate content. Choices from the starch list include cereals, grains, bread, starchy vegetables (peas, corn, yams), and cooked dried beans, peas, and lentils. In general, one starch serving is ½ cup of cereal, pasta, or starchy vegetable, or one 1-ounce (28-g) slice of bread. The fruit list contains fresh, frozen, canned, and dried fruits; one serving is usually one small to medium-size fruit or ½ cup (120 ml) fruit juice. The milk list includes different types of milk and yogurt. Each serving contains the same amount of carbohydrate and protein, but the amount of fat varies depending on whether you choose skim (nonfat), low-fat, or whole milk. A serving of milk is 1 cup (8 fluid ounces/240 ml) or ¾ cup (180 ml) yogurt.

The *meat and meat substitutes group* lists very lean, lean, medium-fat, and high-fat foods rich in animal or vegetable protein. This group contains a consistent amount of protein per serving, but the fat varies from the very lean to the high-fat list depending on the amount of fat. Some examples of animal protein are meat, poultry, fish, or cheese; the serving size is 1 ounce (28 g) cooked. Servings of vegetable protein include ½ cup tofu (4 ounces/115 g) and ½ cup cooked dried beans, peas, or lentils, which are also listed in the carbohydrate group because they contain 15 grams of carbohydrate per serving. Vegetarians tend to count dried cooked beans, peas, and lentils as a protein source in their meal plans.

All fats in the *fat group* contain the same number of fat grams per serving. In the complete Exchange Lists for Meal Planning, the fat group lists foods based on the main type of fatty acids they contain: monounsaturated, polyunsaturated, or saturated. Choices from the monounsaturated list are avocados, olives, almonds, and peanuts; and canola, olive, and peanut oil. Choices from the polyunsaturated list are margarine and mayonnaise; and corn, safflower, and soybean oil. Choices from the

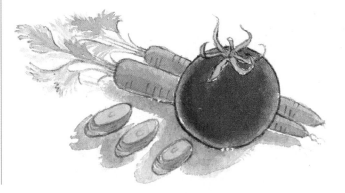

EXCHANGE LISTS FOR MEAL PLANNING

GROUPS/LISTS (per serving)	CARBOHYDRATE (grams)	PROTEIN (grams)	FAT (grams)	CALORIES
Carbohydrate				
Starch	15	3	trace	80
Fruit	15	0	0	60
Milk				
Skim (nonfat)	12	8	0–3	90
Low-fat	12	8	5	120
Whole	12	8	8	150
Other carbohydrates	15	varies	varies	varies
Vegetables (nonstarchy)	5	2	0	25
Meat and Meat Substitutes				
Very lean	0	7	0–1	35
Lean	0	7	3	55
Medium-fat	0	7	5	75
High-fat	0	7	8	100
Fat				
Fat	0	0	5	45

To order the complete Exchange Lists for Meal Planning, call the American Dietetic Association at 1 (800) 745-0775; or call the American Diabetes Association at 1 (800) 232-3472.

saturated list are bacon, butter, coconut, cream cheese, and sour cream. In general, one fat serving is 1 teaspoon of regular margarine or vegetable oil.

FOOD LABELS

As you grocery shop, let the standardized labels now required on all canned and packaged goods help you make healthful food choices. Under the heading "Nutrition Facts" on the label, you'll find information on calories per serving and calories from fat, followed by a listing of amounts of total fat, saturated fat, cholesterol, sodium, total carbohydrate (including dietary fiber and sugars), and protein. Immedi-ately beneath the heading, you'll also find the serving size (in both United States standard measures and metric equivalents) and the number of servings per container. It's important to check the serving sizes carefully, since the portion sizes for some packaged goods may not match the portion size of a Food Exchange.

When you prepare meals from the *Sunset Diabetic Cookbook*, you should refer to the nutritional data provided with each recipe just as you would a food label: The data gives you the facts you need—both Food Exchange information and an extensive nutrient analysis—to devise a healthy eating plan. (See A Word About Our Nutritional Data, page 8.)

MEAL PLANNING

There is no one diet for people with diabetes. For many years, nutrition experts thought that sucrose (table sugar) and sugar-containing foods (sweets) raised blood glucose too quickly and were therefore impermissible in a diabetic diet. But these old beliefs don't stand up to recent research. The American Diabetes Association's recently revised "Nutrition Guidelines and Principles for People with Diabetes," published in May 1994 (*Diabetes Care* 17: 490–522), focuses on an individualized diet that promotes optimal blood glucose and blood lipid control. The revised guidelines include the following recommendations:

Include sufficient calories in your meals to promote a healthy body weight. If you are overweight, marked improvements in blood glucose levels can be achieved with a modest weight reduction of 10 to 20 pounds (4.5 to 9.1 kg). To keep the blood glucose level within an acceptable range, the amount of food you eat and when you eat it must match your medication and physical activity schedules. Choose a commercial weight-control program only after consulting your health-care team.

Select protein-rich foods from a variety of animal and plant sources. Animal proteins include lean meat, fish, poultry, cheese, and eggs; plant proteins are found in dried beans, nuts, and soy products. Trim excess fat from meat, fish, and poultry; limit consumption of higher-fat products such as bacon and sausage. With regard to required amounts of protein, people with diabetes need the same quantity per day as does the general population.

Choose fat-containing foods with care. People with diabetes have an increased risk of cardiovascular disease. Keep saturated fat, found in all animal products and some plant products (coconut and palm oils), to less than 10 percent of the day's total calories. Limit cholesterol (found only in animal products) to less than 300 milligrams per day. Choose vegetable oils and table spreads rich in monounsaturated and polyunsaturated fatty acids (for examples of these, see the discussion under "Exchange Lists for Meal Planning," pages 4–6). When selecting foods containing animal fats, use nutrition labels to help identify those that are lower in saturated fat and cholesterol. Opt for low-fat and nonfat dairy products; as noted previously, be sure to trim all excess fat from meat, poultry, and fish.

Include moderate amounts of carbohydrate-rich foods in your meal plan. Carbohydrates are composed of sugars and starches; for your plan, select foods such as bread, pasta, rice, cereal, fruits, and vegetables. Because sugars and starches have the same effect on blood glucose, you'll have to decide—with the help of your dietitian—how to create a balance. For instance, if your meal plan calls for a sandwich

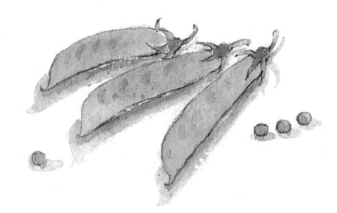

and a serving of fruit, you can replace the fruit, which contains 15 grams of carbohydrate, with a small cookie containing the same amount of carbohydrate.

For assistance in developing a meal plan that will meet your specific calorie and nutrient needs for diabetes control, consult a registered dietitian (R.D.). Your plan can be designed using your favorite ethnic foods and the recipes in this book, allowing you plenty of flexibility, appetite satisfaction—and optimal blood glucose and blood lipid control. To contact an R.D. in your area, call the American Dietetic Association, Consumer Nutrition Hot Line at 1 (800) 366-1655.

DIETARY GUIDELINES

Yes, the USDA Dietary Guidelines for Americans are for people with diabetes, too! Daily use of these guidelines encourages a balanced diet and healthful eating habits through: Eating a variety of foods; balancing the food you eat with physical activity to maintain or improve your weight; choosing a diet with plenty of grain products, vegetables, and fruits; choosing a diet low in fat, saturated fat, and cholesterol; choosing a diet moderate in sugars; choosing a diet moderate in salt and sodium; and, for those who drink alcoholic beverages, drinking in moderation. All the recipes in this book support these guidelines.

DIABETES & EXERCISE

Physical activity is encouraged for most people with diabetes, since it can lower blood glucose levels and help maintain a healthy weight. To avoid dangerous drops in blood glucose (hypoglycemia), it's important to monitor levels before and after exercise. Before starting an exercise regimen, work with your health-care team to establish guidelines to match exercise with blood glucose and food intake. As a general rule, blood glucose should be kept between 80 and 150 mg/dl while you exercise. The amount of carbohydrate needed to cover the exercise is determined by the individual's body weight and by the intensity and duration of the exercise. The guidelines you and your team devise will help you decide when you need a snack to control blood glucose as you exercise.

Ann M. Coulston, M.S., R.D., Senior Research Dietitian
Patricia M. Schaaf, M.S., R.D., C.D.E.
Certified Diabetes Educator
Stanford University Hospital, General Clinical Research Center

A WORD ABOUT OUR NUTRITIONAL DATA

For our recipes, we provide information on the following Food Exchanges: starch, fruit, milk, other carbohydrates, vegetables, meat/protein, and fat. We also provide a nutritional analysis stating calorie count; percentage of calories from fat; grams of total fat and saturated fat; milligrams of cholesterol and sodium; grams of carbohydrates, fiber, and protein; and milligrams of calcium and iron.

Generally, both the Food Exchanges and the nutritional analysis apply to a single serving, based on the number of servings given for each recipe and the amount of each ingredient. If a range is given for the amount of an ingredient, the analysis is based on the average of the figures given. The analysis does not include optional ingredients or those for which no specific amount is stated. If an ingredient is listed with a substitution, the information was calculated using the first choice.

❖ Soups ❖

Warm-Up Vegetable Soup

PREPARATION TIME About 25 minutes • **COOKING TIME** About 40 minutes

S tart off a casual cool-weather supper with bowls of com-
forting vegetable soup. An herb-scented chicken broth
surrounds pasta shells and a colorful medley of mushrooms,
potato chunks, squash, and tomatoes.

1 Heat oil in a 5- to 6-quart (5- to 6-liter) pan over medium
heat. Add onion, mushrooms, oregano, basil, and marjoram.
Cook, stirring often, until vegetables are tinged with brown
(about 10 minutes). Stir in broth, potato, and squash. Bring
to a boil; reduce heat, cover, and boil gently until potato is
tender to bite (about 15 minutes).

2 Add pasta, cover, and continue to cook until pasta is just
tender to bite (10 to 12 minutes). Stir in tomatoes; simmer
until heated through (about 2 minutes). Season to taste with
salt and pepper.

**1 tablespoon (15 ml) olive oil or
vegetable oil**

**1 medium-size onion (about 6 oz./170 g),
finely chopped**

8 ounces (230 g) mushrooms, thinly sliced

1 teaspoon dried oregano

1 teaspoon dried basil

1 teaspoon dried marjoram

**6 cups (1.4 liters) fat-free reduced-sodium
chicken broth**

**1 medium-size thin-skinned potato
(about 6 oz./170 g), peeled and cut
into ½-inch (1-cm) cubes**

**1 pound (455 g) banana squash, peeled
and cut into ½-inch (1-cm) cubes**

**¾ cup (85 g) dried small shell-shaped
pasta**

**1 cup (155 g) diced pear-shaped (Roma-
type) tomatoes**

Salt and pepper

P E R   S E R V I N G

E X C H A N G E S
1¼ starch, 0 fruit, 0 milk,
0 other carbohydrates/sugar, 1½ vegetables,
0 meat/protein, 1 fat

N U T R I E N T S
165 calories (26% calories from fat), 6 g total fat,
1 g saturated fat, 0 mg cholesterol,
126 mg sodium, 27 g carbohydrates, 3 g fiber,
8 g protein, 46 mg calcium, 2 mg iron

M A K E S   6   S E R V I N G S

9

Garlic Soup with Ravioli

PREPARATION TIME About 20 minutes • **COOKING TIME** About 35 minutes

1 head garlic

1 teaspoon olive oil or vegetable oil

6 cups (1.4 liters) fat-free reduced-sodium chicken broth

1 package (about 9 oz./255 g) fresh low-fat cheese ravioli or tortellini

3 tablespoons finely chopped red bell pepper

3 tablespoons thinly sliced green onions

¼ teaspoon dark Oriental sesame oil (optional)

Cilantro

Long popular as a seasoning, garlic is now showing up more and more as a principal ingredient, as in this light soup. Slow cooking tones down the garlic's assertiveness, and the addition of pasta balances the dish.

1 Peel garlic; thinly slice cloves. Heat olive oil in a nonstick frying pan over medium-low heat. Add garlic and cook, stirring often, until golden brown (about 10 minutes; do not scorch). If pan appears dry or garlic sticks to pan bottom, stir in water, 1 tablespoon (15 ml) at a time.

2 Meanwhile, bring broth to a boil in a 4- to 5-quart (3.8- to 5-liter) pan over high heat. When garlic is done, pour about ½ cup (120 ml) of the broth into frying pan, stirring to loosen browned bits. Return garlic mixture to broth; reduce heat, cover, and simmer for 15 minutes.

3 Increase heat to high and bring to a boil. Separate any ravioli that have stuck together; add pasta to broth. Reduce heat and boil gently, stirring occasionally, just until pasta is tender to bite (4 to 6 minutes; or according to package directions).

4 Add bell pepper, onions, and, if desired, sesame oil, and cook just until heated through (about 2 minutes). Garnish with cilantro.

PER SERVING

EXCHANGES
1¼ starch, 0 fruit, 0 milk,
0 other carbohydrates/sugar, 1 vegetable,
½ medium-fat meat/protein, ½ fat

NUTRIENTS
164 calories (28% calories from fat), 6 g total fat,
2 g saturated fat, 26 mg cholesterol,
268 mg sodium, 23 g carbohydrates, 1 g fiber,
10 g protein, 111 mg calcium, 1 mg iron

MAKES 6 SERVINGS

Garlic Soup with Ravioli ▶

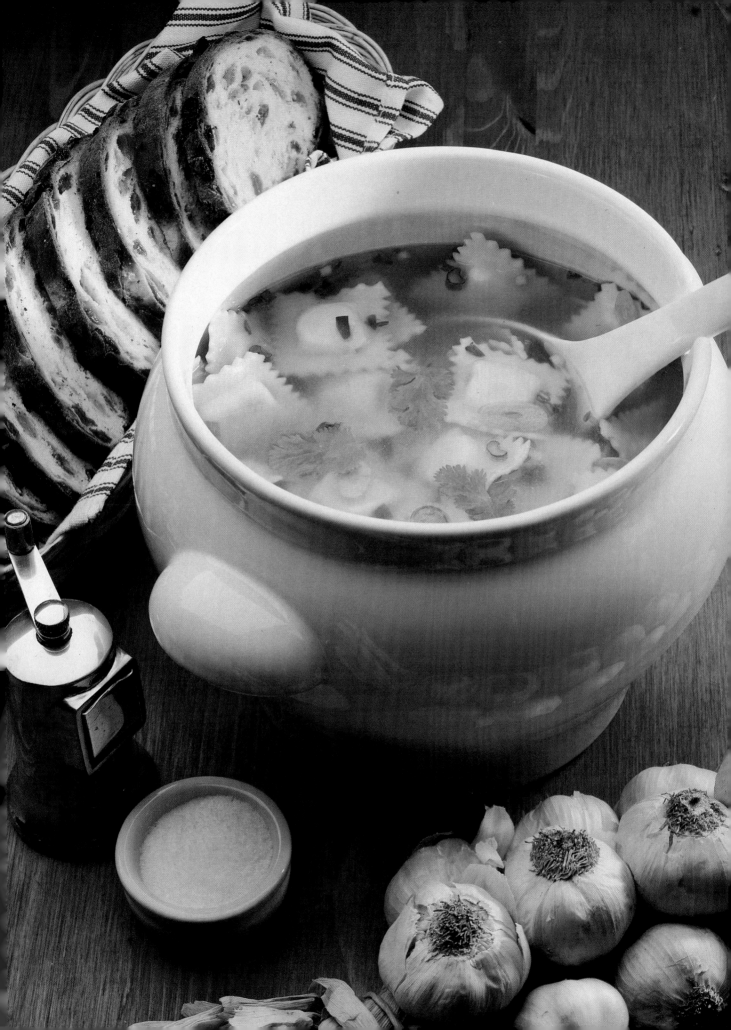

Black & White Bean Soup

1 large onion (about 8 oz./230 g), chopped

1 clove garlic, peeled and sliced

½ cup (120 ml) water

3½ cups (830 ml) fat-free reduced-sodium chicken broth

⅓ cup (55 g) drained oil-packed dried tomatoes, minced

4 green onions (about 2 oz./55 g total), thinly sliced

¼ cup (60 ml) dry sherry

2 cans (about 15 oz./425 g each) black beans, drained and rinsed; or 4 cups (665 g) cooked black beans, drained and rinsed

2 cans (about 15 oz./425 g each) cannellini (white kidney beans), drained and rinsed; or 4 cups (740 g) cooked cannellini, drained and rinsed

Slivered green onions (optional)

Striking to look at, this first-course soup features black and white bean purées, poured side by side into each bowl for a two-tone effect.

1 In a 5- to 6-quart (5- to 6-liter) pan, combine chopped onion, garlic, and water. Cook over high heat, stirring often, until liquid evaporates and onion begins to brown. To deglaze, add 2 tablespoons (30 ml) of the broth; stir to scrape browned bits free. Continue to cook, stirring occasionally, until mixture begins to brown again. Add 2 more tablespoons (30 ml) broth; stir to scrape browned bits free. Stir in ½ cup (120 ml) more broth; pour mixture into a food processor or blender.

2 In same pan, combine tomatoes and sliced green onions. Stir over high heat until onions are wilted (about 2 minutes). Add sherry and cook, stirring, until liquid has evaporated. Remove from heat.

3 To onion mixture in food processor, add black beans. Whirl, gradually adding 1¼ cups (300 ml) of the broth, until smooth. Pour into a 3- to 4-quart (2.8- to 3.8-liter) pan.

4 Rinse processor; add cannellini and whirl until smooth, gradually adding remaining 1½ cups (360 ml) broth. Stir puréed cannellini into pan with tomato mixture. Place both pans of soup over medium-high heat and cook, stirring often, until steaming.

5 To serve, pour soup into 6 bowls as follows: From pans (or from 2 lipped containers such as 1-quart/950-ml pitchers, which are easier to handle), pour soups simultaneously into opposite sides of each wide 1½- to 2-cup (360- to 470-ml) soup bowl so that soups flow together but do not mix. Garnish with slivered green onions, if desired.

PER SERVING

EXCHANGES
1½ starch, 0 fruit, 0 milk,
¼ other carbohydrates/sugar,
2½ vegetables, 0 meat/protein, 2 fat

NUTRIENTS
298 calories (28% calories from fat),
10 g total fat, 2 g saturated fat, 0 mg cholesterol,
482 mg sodium, 38 g carbohydrates, 11 g fiber,
16 g protein, 91 mg calcium, 4 mg iron

MAKES 6 SERVINGS

Caribbean Corn Chowder

PREPARATION TIME About 15 minutes • **COOKING TIME** About 15 minutes

This mellow soup can be served hot or cool and is equally good as a starter or a simple entrée. Fresh chiles add a pleasantly spicy accent to the broth.

1 Heat oil in a 5- to 6-quart (5- to 6-liter) pan over medium-high heat. Add onion, bell pepper, and chiles. Cook, stirring often, until onion is soft (about 5 minutes). Add broth, minced tarragon, and pepper; bring to a boil.

2 Meanwhile, cut corn kernels from cobs. Add corn to boiling broth mixture. Reduce heat, cover, and simmer until corn is hot, about 5 minutes. (At this point, you may let cool; then cover and refrigerate for up to 1 day.) Serve hot or cool.

3 To serve, ladle soup into bowls; garnish with tarragon sprigs, if desired.

1 tablespoon (15 ml) olive oil or vegetable oil

1 large onion (about 8 oz./230 g), finely chopped

1 large red, yellow, or green bell pepper (about 8 oz./230 g), seeded and chopped

3 large fresh green Anaheim or other large mild chiles (about 8 oz./230 g total), seeded and chopped

5½ cups (1.3 liters) fat-free reduced-sodium chicken broth

2 tablespoons minced fresh tarragon or 1 teaspoon dried tarragon

¼ teaspoon pepper

5 large ears corn (about 3½ lbs./1.6 kg total), husks and silk removed

Tarragon sprigs (optional)

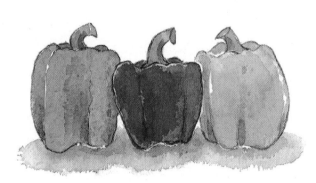

P E R   S E R V I N G

E X C H A N G E S
1½ starch, 0 fruit, 0 milk,
0 other carbohydrates/sugar, 1 vegetable,
0 meat/protein, 1 fat

N U T R I E N T S
159 calories (27% calories from fat), 6 g total fat,
1 g saturated fat, 0 mg cholesterol,
124 mg sodium, 28 g carbohydrates, 5 g fiber,
7 g protein, 36 mg calcium, 1 mg iron

M A K E S   6   S E R V I N G S

Fish Pot-au-Feu

5 cups (1.2 liters) fat-free reduced-sodium chicken broth

1 cup (240 ml) dry white wine; or 1 cup (240 ml) fat-free reduced-sodium chicken broth plus 3 tablespoons (45 ml) white wine vinegar

½ teaspoon dried tarragon

4 small red thin-skinned potatoes (each 1½ to 2 inches/3.5 to 5 cm in diameter), scrubbed

4 medium-size carrots (about 10 oz./ 285 g total), halved

4 medium-size leeks (about 2 lbs./ 905 g total)

1½ pounds (680 g) firm-textured white-fleshed fish fillets such as lingcod or sea bass

Lemon wedges

A classic pot-au-feu simmers slowly for several hours, but this quick contemporary version delivers equally rich flavor after just half an hour. Each bowlful offers carrot and leek halves, a tiny whole potato, and mild, firm fish. For colorful, crunchy contrast, accompany the soup with a salad made with radicchio or red cabbage.

1 In a 5- to 6-quart (5- to 6-liter) pan, combine broth, wine, and tarragon; bring to a boil over high heat. Add potatoes and carrots; return to a boil. Then reduce heat, cover, and boil gently for 10 minutes.

2 Meanwhile, trim ends and all but 3 inches (8 cm) of green tops from leeks; remove tough outer leaves. Split leeks lengthwise; rinse well. Add leeks to pan, cover, and boil gently until leeks and potatoes are tender when pierced (about 10 more minutes). Lift leeks from broth with a slotted spoon, cover, and keep warm.

3 Rinse fish and pat dry; then cut into 4 equal portions. Add fish to soup, cover, and simmer until carrots are tender when pierced and fish is just opaque but still moist in thickest part; cut to test (7 to 10 minutes).

4 With a slotted spatula, carefully lift fish from pan and arrange in 4 wide, shallow bowls. Evenly distribute vegetables alongside fish and ladle broth over all. Serve the soup with lemon wedges.

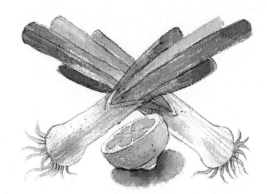

PER SERVING

EXCHANGES
¾ starch, 0 fruit, 0 milk,
0 other carbohydrates/sugar, 3½ vegetables,
4 very lean meat/protein, 1 fat

NUTRIENTS
308 calories (15% calories from fat), 5 g total fat,
1 g saturated fat, 89 mg cholesterol,
296 mg sodium, 33 g carbohydrates, 4 g fiber,
37 g protein, 130 mg calcium, 4 mg iron

MAKES 4 SERVINGS

Tuna Bean Chowder

‣◦

PREPARATION TIME About 15 minutes • **COOKING TIME** About 30 minutes

Keep this chowder in mind for a busy weeknight. It's quickly assembled with staples from the kitchen cupboard: canned tuna, two kinds of beans, and tomatoes.

1 In a 5- to 6-quart (5- to 6-liter) pan, combine chopped onion and mushrooms. Cover and cook over medium-high heat until vegetables release their liquid (5 to 8 minutes). Uncover. Bring to a boil over high heat; then boil, stirring often, until liquid evaporates and vegetables begin to brown. To deglaze, add ¼ cup (60 ml) of the broth and stir to scrape browned bits free. Continue to cook, stirring occasionally, until vegetables begin to brown again.

2 Add pinto and kidney beans to pan; then add remaining 4¾ cups (1.1 liters) broth, tomatoes, tomato sauce, and oregano. Stir to combine. Bring to a boil over high heat; then reduce heat, cover, and simmer for 15 minutes. (At this point, you may let cool, then cover and refrigerate for up to 1 day. Reheat before continuing.)

3 Stir tuna into soup; heat through. Ladle soup into bowls and top with green onions, if desired.

1 large onion (8 oz./230 g), chopped

4 ounces (115 g) mushrooms, sliced

5 cups (1.2 liters) fat-free reduced-sodium chicken broth

2 cans (about 15 oz./425 g each) pinto beans, drained and rinsed; or 4 cups (555 g) cooked pinto beans, drained and rinsed

2 cans (about 15 oz./425 g each) red kidney beans, drained and rinsed; or 4 cups (740 g) cooked red kidney beans, drained and rinsed

1 large can (about 28 oz./795 g) chopped tomatoes

1 can (about 8 oz./230 g) tomato sauce

½ teaspoon dried oregano

2 cans (about 6 oz./170 g each) water-packed albacore tuna, drained

Thinly sliced green onions (optional)

P E R   S E R V I N G

E X C H A N G E S
1½ starch, 0 fruit, 0 milk,
0 other carbohydrates/sugar, 1¼ vegetables,
1¼ very lean meat/protein, ½ fat

N U T R I E N T S
220 calories (14% calories from fat), 4 g total fat,
0.8 g saturated fat, 15 mg cholesterol,
772 mg sodium, 29 g carbohydrates, 8 g fiber,
21 g protein, 82 mg calcium, 3 mg iron

M A K E S   9   S E R V I N G S

Chicken, Shiitake & Bok Choy Soup

PREPARATION TIME About 25 minutes • **COOKING TIME** About 35 minutes

¾ cup (85 g) coarsely chopped fresh ginger

3 cloves garlic, peeled

3 tablespoons (45 ml) seasoned rice vinegar (or 3 tablespoons/45 ml distilled white vinegar plus 1 tablespoon sugar)

1½ tablespoons (23 ml) Oriental sesame oil or olive oil

5 to 6 ounces (140 to 170 g) fresh shiitake or regular mushrooms, thinly sliced

8 green onions (about 4 oz./115 g total), sliced

3 cups (710 ml) fat-free reduced-sodium chicken broth

4 skinless, boneless chicken breast halves (about 1½ lbs./680 g total)

2 large carrots (about 7 oz./200 g total), cut into thin diagonal slices

8 baby bok choy (about 12 oz./340 g total), coarse outer leaves removed

2 cups (260 g) hot cooked short- or medium-grain rice

3 tablespoons minced cilantro

Too pretty to eat? Almost, but this combination of tender-crisp vegetables, rice, and chicken in a clear broth is too tempting to resist. A bold ginger-garlic paste, passed at the table, gives each bowlful a flavor boost.

1 To prepare ginger-garlic paste, in a blender or food processor, combine ginger, garlic, and vinegar. Whirl until very smooth. Spoon into a small bowl and set aside. (At this point, you may cover and refrigerate for up to 4 hours.) Makes about ½ cup (120 ml).

2 Heat oil in a 4- to 5-quart (3.8- to 5-liter) pan over medium heat. Add mushrooms and half the onions; cook, stirring often, until mushrooms are lightly browned (about 10 minutes). Add broth and stir to scrape browned bits free. Cover pan and bring broth to a boil over high heat.

3 Rinse chicken; pat dry. Add chicken and carrots to boiling broth, making sure meat and vegetables are covered with liquid. Reduce heat to low, cover, and simmer until meat in thickest part of chicken breasts is no longer pink; cut to test (about 15 minutes).

4 Lift chicken to a cutting board. Add bok choy and remaining onions to pan; cover and simmer over medium heat until bok choy is bright green and just tender when pierced (about 5 minutes). Meanwhile, cut chicken across the grain into ½-inch-wide (1-cm-wide) diagonal slices.

5 Place a ½-cup scoop (65-g) of rice off center in each of 4 wide, shallow soup bowls. Arrange a sliced chicken breast around each mound of rice. With a slotted spoon, distribute vegetables evenly among bowls. Stir cilantro into broth; then gently pour broth into bowls over chicken and vegetables. Offer ginger-garlic paste to stir into soup to taste.

PER SERVING

EXCHANGES
1¾ starch, 0 fruit, 0 milk,
0 other carbohydrates/sugar, 3 vegetables,
4½ very lean meat/protein, 2 fat

NUTRIENTS
436 calories (20% calories from fat), 10 g total
fat, 2 g saturated fat, 99 mg cholesterol,
276 mg sodium, 42 g carbohydrates, 4 g fiber,
47 g protein, 159 mg calcium, 5 mg iron

MAKES 4 SERVINGS

Tortellini & Chicken Soup

PREPARATION TIME About 10 minutes • **COOKING TIME** About 15 minutes

Here's a soup with a wide range of ingredients—chicken, rice, vegetables, even cheese-filled spinach pasta. Let diners add Parmesan cheese to taste. If you're concerned about sodium, consider using reduced-sodium chicken broth.

1 In an 8- to 10-quart (8- to 10-liter) pan, bring broth to a boil over high heat. Add tortellini; reduce heat and boil gently, uncovered, until just tender to bite (about 6 minutes).

2 Add spinach, chicken, mushrooms, bell pepper, rice, and tarragon to broth; return to a boil over high heat. Then reduce heat, cover, and simmer until chicken is no longer pink in center; cut to test (about 2 minutes). Season soup to taste with salt and pepper; serve with cheese to add to taste.

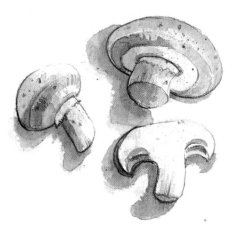

3 large cans (about 49½ oz./1.4 kg each) chicken broth; or 4½ quarts (4.3 liters) homemade chicken broth

1 package (about 9 oz./255 g) fresh cheese-filled spinach tortellini

1 pound (455 g) spinach, stems removed, leaves rinsed and coarsely chopped

1 pound (455 g) skinless, boneless chicken breasts, cut into ½-inch (1-cm) chunks

8 ounces (230 g) mushrooms, sliced

1 medium-size red bell pepper (about 6 oz./170 g), seeded and diced

1 cup (130 g) cooked rice

2 teaspoons dried tarragon

Salt and pepper

Grated Parmesan cheese

PER SERVING

EXCHANGES
1 starch, 0 fruit, 0 milk,
0 other carbohydrates/sugar, ¾ vegetable,
2 lean meat/protein, 0 fat

NUTRIENTS
204 calories (26% calories from fat), 6 g total fat,
1 g saturated fat, 39 mg cholesterol,
1,785 mg sodium, 19 g carbohydrates, 2 g fiber,
18 g protein, 82 mg calcium, 2 mg iron

MAKES 11 SERVINGS

Harvest Turkey Soup

PREPARATION TIME About 20 minutes • **COOKING TIME** About 40 minutes

Vegetable oil cooking spray

1 pound (455 g) ground skinless turkey breast

1 medium-size onion (about 6 oz./170 g), chopped

1 teaspoon dried oregano

1 teaspoon Italian herb seasoning; or ¼ teaspoon each dried basil, dried marjoram, dried oregano, and dried thyme

3 large firm-ripe tomatoes (about 1¼ lbs./565 g total), chopped

3 large carrots (about 10½ oz./300 g total), thinly sliced

1 large potato (about 8 oz./230 g), peeled and diced

6 cups (1.4 liters) beef broth

1 cup (240 ml) tomato juice

1 cup (240 ml) dry red wine

1 tablespoon (15 ml) Worcestershire

½ cup (55 g) dried tiny pasta bow ties (tripolini) or other small shapes

2 medium-size zucchini (about 12 oz./ 340 g total), coarsely diced

Liquid hot pepper seasoning

Hearty and warming, this meaty soup includes pasta, fragrant herbs, and plenty of fresh vegetables. Rich beefy flavor is provided by the broth, while fat is kept low with turkey meat. Use the leanest packaged ground turkey you can find (check the label for the fat content); or have the butcher grind turkey breast for you.

1 Coat a wide 4- to 5-quart (3.8- to 5-liter) pan with cooking spray. Crumble turkey into pan; add onion, oregano, and herb seasoning. Cook over medium heat, stirring often, until turkey is no longer pink and onion is soft but not browned (about 5 minutes).

2 Stir in tomatoes, carrots, potato, broth, tomato juice, wine, and Worcestershire. Increase heat to medium-high and bring to a boil; then reduce heat, cover, and boil gently for 20 minutes.

3 Add pasta; cover and cook for 5 minutes. Stir in zucchini and boil gently, uncovered, until pasta and zucchini are just tender to bite (8 to 10 minutes). Season to taste with hot pepper seasoning.

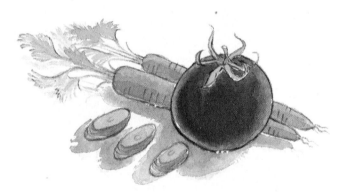

PER SERVING

EXCHANGES
1 starch, 0 fruit, 0 milk, 0 other carbohydrates/sugar, 2½ vegetables, 1½ very lean meat/protein, 1¼ fat

NUTRIENTS
239 calories (25% calories from fat), 7 g total fat, 2 g saturated fat, 47 mg cholesterol, 944 mg sodium, 29 g carbohydrates, 4 g fiber, 18 g protein, 49 mg calcium, 3 mg iron

MAKES 7 SERVINGS

Beef & "Pumpkin" Soup

PREPARATION TIME About 25 minutes • COOKING TIME About 55 minutes

Coarsely mashed Hubbard or banana squash—called "pumpkin" by the islanders of St. Lucia—adds texture to this Caribbean soup. The squash is also an excellent source of vitamin A and contains iron and riboflavin.

1 Heat oil in a 6- to 8-quart (6- to 8-liter) pan over medium-high heat. Add onion and celery; cook, stirring often, until onion is soft (about 5 minutes). Add broth and beef. Bring to a boil; then reduce heat, cover, and simmer for 30 minutes. Add squash and carrots. Bring to a boil; then reduce heat, cover, and simmer until squash and beef are very tender when pierced (about 15 more minutes).

2 With a slotted spoon, lift about three-fourths of the squash from pan; mash coarsely. Return mashed squash to pan, then stir in spinach. Bring to a boil over high heat; then reduce heat and simmer, uncovered, until spinach is wilted (about 3 minutes). Skim and discard fat from soup, if necessary; season soup to taste with salt and pepper.

1 tablespoon (15 ml) olive oil or vegetable oil

1 large onion (about 8 oz./230 g), chopped

1 stalk celery (about 1½ oz./45 g), thinly sliced

8 cups (1.9 liters) fat-free reduced-sodium chicken broth

8 ounces (230 g) boneless beef chuck, trimmed of fat and cut into ½-inch (1-cm) cubes

3½ pounds (1.6 kg) Hubbard or banana squash, peeled, seeded, and cut into ½-inch (1-cm) cubes (you should have about 10 cups)

3 large carrots (about 10½ oz./300 g total), coarsely chopped

8 ounces (230 g) spinach, stems removed, leaves rinsed and cut crosswise into ¼-inch-wide (6-mm-wide) strips

Salt and pepper

PER SERVING

EXCHANGES
1 starch, 0 fruit, 0 milk,
0 other carbohydrates/sugar, 1¼ vegetables,
1 medium-fat meat/protein, ½ fat

NUTRIENTS
179 calories (30% calories from fat), 7 g total fat,
2 g saturated fat, 19 mg cholesterol,
200 mg sodium, 22 g carbohydrates, 5 g fiber,
15 g protein, 83 mg calcium, 2 mg iron

MAKES 7 SERVINGS

Italian Sausage & Bow-Tie Soup

1 pound (455 g) pork tenderloin or boned pork loin, trimmed of fat

¼ cup (60 ml) dry white wine

½ cup (30 g) plus 2 tablespoons chopped parsley

1½ teaspoons crushed fennel seeds

½ teaspoon crushed red pepper flakes

4 cloves garlic, minced or pressed

2 large onions (about 1 lb./455 g total), chopped

5 cups (1.2 liters) beef broth

1 can (about 28 oz./795 g) pear-shaped tomatoes

1½ cups (360 ml) dry red wine

1 tablespoon dried basil

1 tablespoon sugar

1 medium-size green bell pepper (about 6 oz./170 g), seeded and chopped

2 medium-size zucchini (about 8 oz./230 g total), sliced ¼-inch (6-mm) thick

5 ounces/140 g (about 2½ cups) dried farfalle (about 1½-inch/3.5-cm size)

Salt and pepper

PER SERVING

EXCHANGES

1 starch, 0 fruit, 0 milk,
¾ other carbohydrates/sugar, 3 vegetables,
2 very lean meat/protein, 1 fat

NUTRIENTS

327 calories (14% calories from fat), 5 g total fat,
1 g saturated fat, 49 mg cholesterol,
949 mg sodium, 38 g carbohydrates, 4 g fiber,
24 g protein, 103 mg calcium, 4 mg iron

MAKES 6 SERVINGS

Homemade ultra-lean sausage and slow-cooked onions contribute rich flavor but very little fat to this filling soup. The pasta looks like little bow ties; the Italians, though, call these noodles *farfalle*, or "butterflies."

1 To prepare sausage, cut pork tenderloin into 1-inch (2.5-cm) chunks. Whirl in a food processor, half at a time, until coarsely chopped (or put through a food chopper fitted with a medium blade). In a large bowl, combine pork, white wine, 2 tablespoons of the parsley, fennel seeds, red pepper flakes, and half the minced garlic. Mix well. Cover and refrigerate. (At this point, you may refrigerate for up to a day.)

2 Combine onions, remaining garlic, and 1 cup (240 ml) of the broth in a 5- to 6-quart (5- to 6-liter) pan. Bring to a boil over medium-high heat and cook, stirring occasionally, until liquid has evaporated and onion mixture begins to brown (about 10 minutes). To deglaze pan, add 3 tablespoons (45 ml) water, stirring to loosen browned bits. Continue to cook, stirring often, until liquid has evaporated and onion mixture begins to brown again (about 1 minute). Repeat deglazing step, adding 3 tablespoons (45 ml) more water each time, until onion mixture is richly browned.

3 Stir in sausage and ½ cup (120 ml) more water. Cook, stirring gently, until liquid has evaporated and meat begins to brown (8 to 10 minutes).

4 Add remaining 4 cups (950 ml) broth, stirring to loosen browned bits. Stir in tomatoes (breaking up with a spoon) and their liquid, wine, basil, sugar, bell pepper, zucchini, and pasta. Bring to a boil over high heat; reduce heat, cover, and simmer just until pasta is tender to bite (about 15 minutes).

5 Sprinkle soup with remaining ½ cup (30 g) parsley. Offer salt and pepper to add to taste.

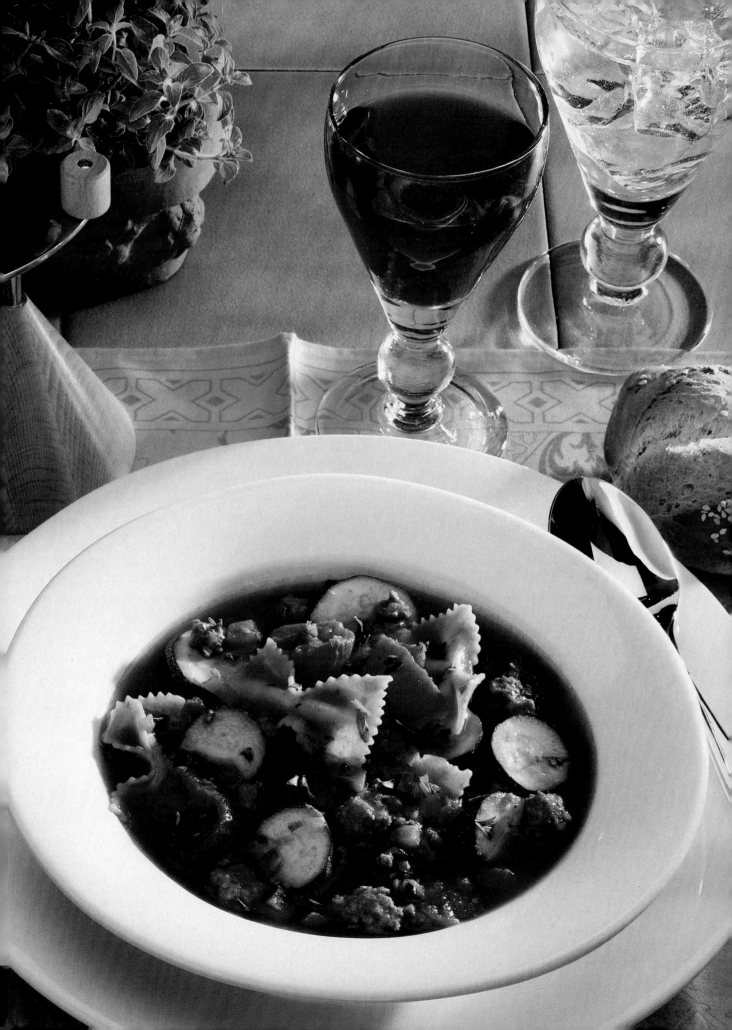

Albóndigas Soup

1½ pounds (680 g) extra-lean ground beef

½ cup (65 g) cooked white or brown rice

¼ cup (30 g) all-purpose flour

¼ cup (60 ml) water

1 teaspoon chili powder

2½ teaspoons ground cumin

1 tablespoon (15 ml) olive oil or vegetable oil

1 large onion (about 8 oz./230 g), cut into slivers

1 teaspoon dried oregano

2 cloves garlic, minced or pressed

1 can (about 14½ oz./415 g) pear-shaped (Roma-type) tomatoes

2 cans (about 14½ oz./415 g each) beef broth

1 large can (about 46 oz./1.3 kg) low-sodium tomato juice

¼ cup (10 g) coarsely chopped cilantro

Salt

Lime wedges

Warm a stack of corn or flour tortillas to serve alongside this colorful Mexican-inspired soup. To keep the rice-studded meatballs low in fat, brown them in the oven instead of frying them.

1 To prepare meatballs with rice, in a large bowl, lightly mix ground beef, rice, flour, water, chili powder, and 1 teaspoon of the cumin. Shape mixture into 1-inch (2.5-cm) balls and place slightly apart in a shallow nonstick baking pan. Bake in a 450°F (230°C) oven until well browned (about 15 minutes). Remove pan from oven; loosen meatballs from baking pan with a wide spatula.

2 While meatballs are baking, heat oil in a 5- to 6-quart (5- to 6-liter) pan over medium heat. Add onion, remaining cumin, and oregano. Cook, stirring often, until onion is golden (6 to 8 minutes); then stir in garlic. Cut up tomatoes; add tomatoes and their liquid, broth, and tomato juice to pan. Bring to a boil over high heat; then reduce heat, cover, and simmer for 15 minutes.

3 Transfer meatballs to soup. Cover and simmer until meatballs are heated through (about 10 minutes). Skim and discard fat from soup, if necessary. Just before serving, stir in cilantro and season to taste with salt. Serve soup with lime wedges.

PER SERVING

EXCHANGES
¾ starch, 0 fruit, 0 milk,
0 other carbohydrates/sugar, 2¾ vegetables,
3 very lean meat/protein, 1½ fat

NUTRIENTS
289 calories (23% calories from fat), 7 g total fat,
2 g saturated fat, 65 mg cholesterol,
678 mg sodium, 26 g carbohydrates, 2 g fiber,
31 g protein, 66 mg calcium, 6 mg iron

MAKES 6 SERVINGS

Pasta & Grapefruit Salad

PREPARATION TIME About 40 minutes • **COOKING TIME** About 5 minutes

Juicy grapefruit segments add a sweet tartness to a salad of tiny pasta bow ties and green peas. Fish sauce gives the dish an Asian flavor.

1 In a 5- to 6-quart (5- to 6-liter) pan, cook pasta in about 3 quarts (2.8 liters) boiling water until just tender to bite (about 5 minutes); or cook according to package directions. Drain, rinse with cold water until cool, and drain again.

2 In a large bowl, combine pasta, peas, celery, onions, and chopped mint.

3 Cut peel and all white membrane from each grapefruit. Holding fruit over a bowl to catch juice, cut between membranes to release grapefruit segments; add segments to pasta mixture. Squeeze membranes over bowl of juice, then measure collected juice; you need about ½ cup (120 ml). Add lemon peel and lemon juice to the ½ cup (120 ml) grapefruit juice. Add juice mixture and chile to pasta mixture; mix gently. Season to taste with fish sauce.

4 To serve, arrange lettuce leaves on 5 individual plates. Spoon pasta salad over lettuce. Roll ham slices and set on plates. Garnish with mint sprigs.

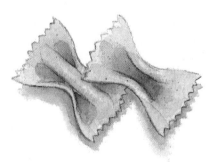

8 ounces (230 g) dried tiny pasta bow ties (tripolini) or other small shapes

1 package (about 1 lb./455 g) frozen tiny peas, thawed

1 cup (120 g) chopped celery

½ cup (50 g) thinly sliced green onions

⅓ cup (15 g) chopped fresh mint

3 large red grapefruit (3 to 3½ lbs./1.35 to 1.6 kg total)

½ teaspoon grated lemon peel

2 tablespoons (30 ml) lemon juice

½ to 1 teaspoon minced fresh hot chile

Fish sauce (*nam pla* or *nuoc mam*) or salt

10 large butter lettuce leaves (about 3½ oz./100 g total), rinsed and crisped

8 ounces (230 g) thinly sliced cooked ham

Mint sprigs

P E R   S E R V I N G

E X C H A N G E S
3 starch, ¾ fruit, 0 milk,
0 other carbohydrates/sugar, ½ vegetable,
1½ lean meat/protein, 0 fat

N U T R I E N T S
366 calories (13% calories from fat), 5 g total fat,
2 g saturated fat, 27 mg cholesterol,
831 mg sodium, 58 g carbohydrates, 6 g fiber,
22 g protein, 64 mg calcium, 4 mg iron

M A K E S   5   S E R V I N G S

Thai Noodle Salad Buffet

PREPARATION TIME About 1 hour • **COOKING TIME** About 10 minutes • **STANDING TIME** About 35 minutes

4 chicken breast halves (about 2 lbs./ 905 g total), skinned

1 pound (455 g) dried angel hair pasta (capellini) or thin rice noodles (*mai fun*)

2 tablespoons (30 ml) plus 2 teaspoons Oriental sesame oil or olive oil

¾ cup (180 ml) unseasoned rice vinegar or white wine vinegar

½ cup (120 ml) reduced-sodium soy sauce

3 tablespoons sugar

2 tablespoons minced fresh ginger

1 to 2 teaspoons crushed red pepper flakes

2 cloves garlic, minced or pressed

1 large English cucumber (about 1 lb./ 455 g), cut into thin slivers

8 to 12 ounces (230 to 340 g) bean sprouts

¾ cup (75 g) thinly sliced green onions

½ cup (20 g) chopped fresh basil

½ cup (72 g) finely chopped salted dry-roasted peanuts

¾ cup (30 g) chopped cilantro

Lemon wedges (optional)

PER SERVING

EXCHANGES
3½ starch, 0 fruit, 0 milk, ½ other carbohydrates/sugar, 3 vegetables, 3 very lean meat/protein, 3 fat

NUTRIENTS
591 calories (23% calories from fat), 15 g total fat, 2 g saturated fat, 57 mg cholesterol, 976 mg sodium, 76 g carbohydrates, 4 g fiber, 39 g protein, 97 mg calcium, 6 mg iron

MAKES 6 SERVINGS

Guests can assemble their own servings of this zesty main dish from an array of fresh and spicy ingredients: crisp vegetables, thin angel hair or Asian rice noodles, shredded chicken, and a gingery sesame dressing. Follow the meal with a dessert of cooling fresh pineapple.

1 In a 5- to 6-quart (5- to 6-liter) pan, bring about 3 quarts (2.8 liters) water to a boil over high heat. Rinse chicken and add to water; return to a boil. Then cover pan tightly, remove from heat, and let stand until meat in thickest part is no longer pink; cut to test (about 20 minutes). If chicken is not done after 20 minutes, return it to water, cover pan, and let stand longer, checking at 2- to 3-minute intervals. Remove chicken from water and let cool; then tear meat into shreds and discard bones.

2 While chicken is cooling, return water to a boil over high heat. Add pasta and cook until just tender to bite (about 3 minutes); or cook according to package directions. Drain, then immerse in a bowl of cold water. Add 2 teaspoons of the oil to water. Let pasta stand until cool (about 15 minutes); then lift pasta from water in small handfuls, draining briefly. Loosely coil each handful of pasta; set coils on a wide platter, stacking if necessary.

3 To prepare spicy sesame dressing, in a small bowl, combine rice vinegar, soy sauce, sugar, remaining 2 tablespoons (30 ml) oil, ginger, red pepper flakes, and garlic. Stir until sugar is completely dissolved.

4 Arrange chicken, cucumber, bean sprouts, onions, and basil in separate groups around pasta on platter. Arrange peanuts, cilantro, and lemon wedges (if using) in small bowls. To assemble each salad, place a few pasta coils on an individual plate. Add other ingredients to taste; spoon on spicy sesame dressing to taste.

Golden Couscous Salad

PREPARATION TIME About 30 minutes • **COOKING TIME** About 3 minutes • **STANDING TIME** About 5 minutes

Orange slices encircle a mound of spiced couscous studded with raisins, crisp cucumber, and green onions in a dish that makes a wonderful, light vegetarian lunch.

1 In a 3- to 4-quart (2.8- to 3.8-liter) pan, bring broth to a boil over high heat. Stir in couscous, raisins, ginger, orange peel, and cumin; cover pan and remove from heat. Let stand until all liquid has been absorbed (about 5 minutes). Fluff couscous lightly with a fork; then stir in vinegar, orange juice, cucumber, and onions. (At this point, you may cover and let stand for up to 4 hours. Stir before using.)

2 Cut peel and all white membrane from oranges; thinly slice oranges crosswise. Arrange orange slices in a ring around edge of a rimmed platter; mound couscous in center. Sprinkle salad with almonds.

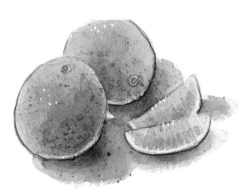

1¼ cups (300 ml) fat-free reduced-sodium chicken broth

1 cup (185 g) couscous

½ cup (75 g) golden raisins

2 tablespoons finely chopped crystallized ginger

1 teaspoon grated orange peel

½ teaspoon ground cumin

3 tablespoons (45 ml) seasoned rice vinegar (or 3 tablespoons/45 ml unseasoned rice vinegar plus 2 teaspoons sugar)

3 tablespoons (45 ml) orange juice

½ cup (72 g) finely chopped cucumber

½ cup (50 g) thinly sliced green onions

4 large oranges (about 2½ lbs./1.15 kg total)

1 to 2 tablespoons chopped salted roasted almonds

P E R   S E R V I N G

E X C H A N G E S
2 starch, 2½ fruit, 0 milk,
0 other carbohydrates/sugar, 0 vegetables,
0 meat/protein, ½ fat

N U T R I E N T S
323 calories (8% calories from fat), 3 g total fat,
0.5 g saturated fat, 0 mg cholesterol,
241 mg sodium, 70 g carbohydrates, 7 g fiber,
8 g protein, 126 mg calcium, 3 mg iron

M A K E S   5   S E R V I N G S

Bean, Corn & Bell Pepper Salad

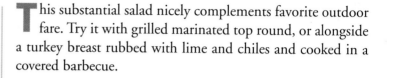

PREPARATION TIME About 15 minutes • **CHILLING TIME** At least 1 hour

2 cans (about 15 oz./425 g each) black beans or cannellini (white kidney beans), drained and rinsed; or 4 cups (665 g) cooked black beans or cannellini, drained and rinsed

1½ cups (174 g) cooked fresh yellow or white corn kernels (from 2 medium-size ears corn); or 1 package (about 10 oz./285 g) frozen corn kernels, thawed

1 large red bell pepper (about 8 oz./ 230 g), seeded and finely chopped

2 small fresh jalapeño chiles, seeded and finely chopped

½ cup (20 g) firmly packed chopped cilantro

¼ cup (60 ml) lime juice

2 tablespoons (30 ml) olive oil

Salt and pepper

Lettuce leaves, rinsed and crisped

This substantial salad nicely complements favorite outdoor fare. Try it with grilled marinated top round, or alongside a turkey breast rubbed with lime and chiles and cooked in a covered barbecue.

1 In a large bowl, combine beans, corn, bell pepper, chiles, cilantro, lime juice, and oil; mix lightly. Season to taste with salt and pepper. Cover and refrigerate for at least 1 hour or for up to 1 day.

2 To serve, line a serving bowl with lettuce leaves; spoon in bean mixture.

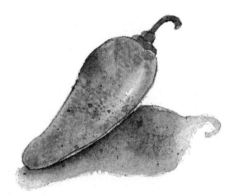

PER SERVING

EXCHANGES
1¾ starch, 0 fruit, 0 milk,
0 other carbohydrates/sugar, ½ vegetable,
0 meat/protein, 1 fat

NUTRIENTS
197 calories (26% calories from fat), 6 g total fat,
0.7 g saturated fat, 0 mg cholesterol,
186 mg sodium, 29 g carbohydrates, 8 g fiber,
9 g protein, 39 mg calcium, 2 mg iron

MAKES 6 SERVINGS

Chili Potato Salad with Chicken

PREPARATION TIME About 15 minutes • **COOKING TIME** 25 to 30 minutes • **COOLING TIME** About 30 minutes

Bored with the same old mayonnaise-drenched potato salad? Offer this lighter chili-flavored version, which also includes chicken, as a light lunch or supper. The salad is tasty cold or at room temperature, but don't let it stand unrefrigerated for more than 2 hours.

1 Place unpeeled potatoes in a 5- to 6-quart (5- to 6-liter) pan and add enough water to cover. Bring to a boil over high heat; then reduce heat, partially cover, and boil gently until potatoes are tender when pierced (25 to 30 minutes). Drain, immerse in cold water until cool, and drain again. Cut into ¾-inch (2-cm) cubes.

2 In a large bowl, combine potatoes, chicken, corn, celery, onion, and bell pepper. Add oil, vinegar, chili powder, garlic, and hot pepper seasoning; mix gently, then season to taste with salt and pepper. (At this point, you may cover and refrigerate for up to 1 day.) Serve cold or at room temperature.

1½ pounds (680 g) large thin-skinned potatoes, scrubbed

12 ounces (340 g) diced cooked chicken breast

1 can (about 17 oz./480 g) corn kernels, drained

½ cup (60 g) sliced celery

½ cup (85 g) chopped red onion

⅔ cup (100 g) chopped red bell pepper

2 tablespoons (30 ml) olive oil

¼ cup (60 ml) cider vinegar

2 teaspoons chili powder

1 clove garlic, minced or pressed

½ teaspoon liquid hot pepper seasoning

Salt and pepper

P E R   S E R V I N G

E X C H A N G E S
2 starch, 0 fruit, 0 milk,
0 other carbohydrates/sugar, ½ vegetable,
2 very lean meat/protein, 1½ fat

N U T R I E N T S
210 calories (21% calories from fat), 5 g total fat,
0.6 g saturated fat, 0 mg cholesterol,
257 mg sodium, 40 g carbohydrates, 4 g fiber,
5 g protein, 17 mg calcium, 1 mg iron

M A K E S   6   S E R V I N G S

Artichokes with Shrimp & Cilantro Salsa

½ cup (120 ml) seasoned rice vinegar (or ½ cup/120 ml distilled white vinegar plus 1 tablespoon sugar)

1 tablespoon mustard seeds

1 teaspoon whole black peppercorns

4 thin quarter-size slices fresh ginger

3 large artichokes (about 12 oz./340 g each), each 4 to 4½ inches (10 to 11 cm) in diameter

12 ounces (340 g) tiny cooked shrimp

⅓ cup (55 g) minced pickled scallions

¼ cup (10 g) minced cilantro

¼ cup (10 g) minced fresh mint or 1 tablespoon dried mint

2 tablespoons (30 ml) reduced-sodium soy sauce

¼ to ½ teaspoon chili oil

Mint or cilantro sprigs

Big artichoke halves filled with a spicy shrimp and cilantro "salsa" make an attractive first course. Pickled scallions, available in well-stocked supermarkets and Asian markets, add a sweet crunch to the salsa.

1 In a 6- to 8-quart (6- to 8-liter) pan, combine ¼ cup (60 ml) of the vinegar, mustard seeds, peppercorns, ginger, and 4 quarts (3.8 liters) water. Cover and bring to a boil over high heat.

2 Meanwhile, remove coarse outer leaves from artichokes and trim stems flush with bases. With a sharp knife, cut off top third of each artichoke. With scissors, trim thorny tips from remaining leaves. Immerse artichokes in cold water and swish back and forth vigorously to release debris; then lift artichokes from water and shake briskly to drain.

3 Lower artichokes into boiling vinegar-water mixture. Then reduce heat and simmer, covered, until artichoke bottoms are tender when pierced (about 35 minutes). Drain, reserving cooking liquid. Let artichokes stand until they are cool enough to handle.

4 Pour artichoke cooking liquid through a fine strainer set over a bowl; discard ginger and reserve mustard seeds and peppercorns. Place shrimp in strainer. Rinse shrimp with cool water; then drain well, place in a bowl, and mix with reserved seasonings, remaining ¼ cup (60 ml) vinegar, scallions, minced cilantro, minced mint, soy sauce, and chili oil. (At this point, you may cover and refrigerate artichokes and shrimp mixture separately until next day.)

5 With a sharp knife, cut each artichoke in half lengthwise. Remove sharp-pointed inner leaves and scoop out fuzzy centers. Set each artichoke half on a salad plate. Spoon shrimp mixture equally into artichokes; garnish with mint sprigs.

PER SERVING

EXCHANGES
0 starch, 0 fruit, 0 milk,
0 other carbohydrates/sugar, 2½ vegetables,
1½ very lean meat/protein, ¼ fat

NUTRIENTS
122 calories (11% calories from fat), 3 g total fat,
0.2 g saturated fat, 111 mg cholesterol,
911 mg sodium, 13 g carbohydrates, 4 g fiber,
15 g protein, 67 mg calcium, 3 mg iron

MAKES 6 SERVINGS

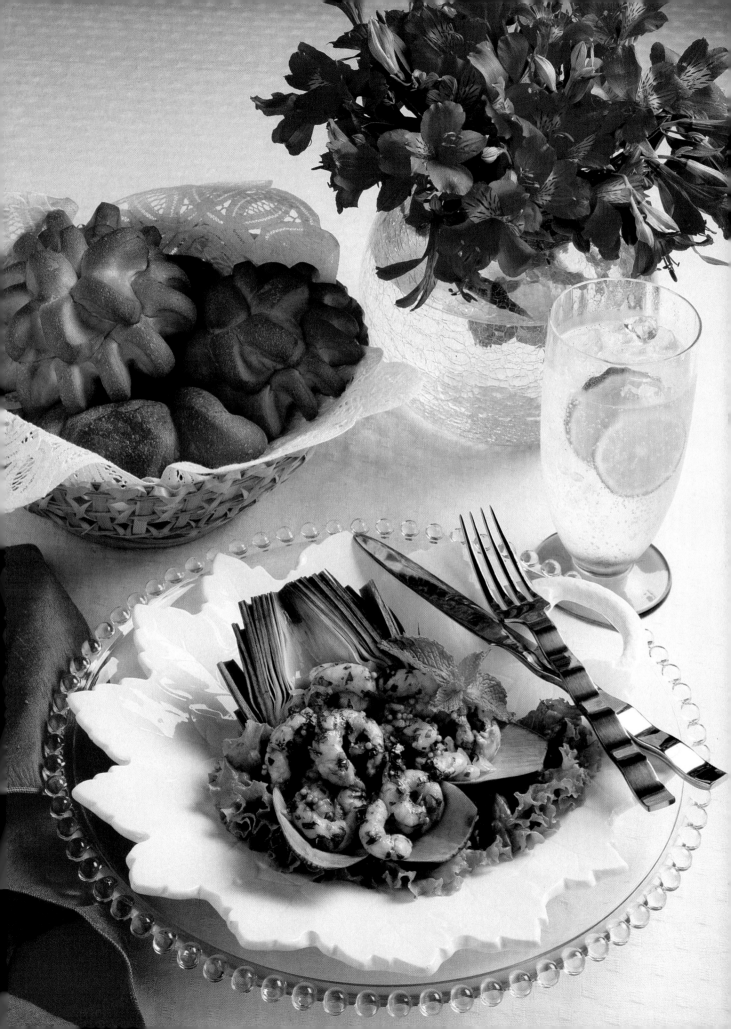

Shrimp & Jicama with Chile Vinegar

PREPARATION TIME About 35 minutes

⅔ cup (160 ml) white wine vinegar

¼ cup (50 g) sugar

2 to 3 tablespoons seeded and minced
fresh hot green chiles

3 to 4 tablespoons chopped cilantro

2 cups (260 g) shredded jicama

1 pound (455 g) small cooked shrimp

4 large ripe tomatoes (about 2 lbs./
905 g total), sliced

4 large tomatillos (about 12 oz./
340 g total), husked, rinsed, and sliced

Cilantro sprigs

Enjoy a taste of Mexico with this main-dish combination of shrimp, tomatillos, and crisp, fruity jicama. The oil-free dressing is hot and full of flavor.

1 To prepare chile vinegar, in a small bowl, stir together vinegar, sugar, chiles, and chopped cilantro.

2 Place jicama and shrimp in separate bowls. Add ¼ cup (60 ml) of the chile vinegar to each bowl; mix gently. Reserve remaining vinegar.

3 On each of 4 individual plates, arrange tomatoes and tomatillos, overlapping slices slightly. Mound jicama over or beside tomato slices. Spoon shrimp over jicama; spoon remaining chile vinegar over all. Garnish with cilantro sprigs.

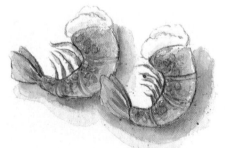

PER SERVING

EXCHANGES
0 starch, 0 fruit, 0 milk,
¾ other carbohydrates/sugar, 4 vegetables,
3 very lean meat/protein, ½ fat

NUTRIENTS
261 calories (8% calories from fat), 3 g total fat,
0.4 g saturated fat, 221 mg cholesterol,
279 mg sodium, 34 g carbohydrates, 4 g fiber,
28 g protein, 73 mg calcium, 5 mg iron

MAKES 4 SERVINGS

Spinach & Shrimp Salad

⬤-⬤

PREPARATION TIME *About 20 minutes* • **COOKING TIME** *About 3 minutes*

The ever-popular wilted spinach and bacon salad provided the inspiration for this recipe. But our salad is considerably leaner than the traditional dish: shrimp replace the bacon, and the delicious warm mustard dressing is prepared without fat.

1 Cut spinach leaves into ½-inch (1-cm) strips, then place in a wide, shallow bowl and top with shrimp. (At this point, you may cover and refrigerate for up to 4 hours.)

2 In a 1- to 1½-quart (950 ml- to 1.4-liter) pan, blend cornstarch and sugar. Stir in vinegar, broth, and mustard. Bring to a boil over high heat, stirring; then stir in dill. Pour hot dressing over salad; mix gently and serve immediately.

12 cups (340 g) firmly packed stemmed spinach leaves, rinsed and crisped

12 ounces (340 g) small cooked shrimp

1 teaspoon cornstarch

1 tablespoon sugar

1 tablespoon (15 ml) unseasoned rice vinegar

¼ cup (60 ml) fat-free reduced-sodium chicken broth or water

⅓ cup (80 ml) Dijon mustard

2 tablespoons minced fresh dill or 1½ teaspoons dried dill weed

P E R   S E R V I N G

E X C H A N G E S
0 starch, 0 fruit, 0 milk,
0 other carbohydrates/sugar, 3 vegetables,
3 very lean meat/protein, ½ fat

N U T R I E N T S
186 calories (10% calories from fat), 2 g total fat,
0.5 g saturated fat, 166 mg cholesterol,
906 mg sodium, 14 g carbohydrates, 8 g fiber,
26 g protein, 332 mg calcium, 11 mg iron

M A K E S   4   S E R V I N G S

Mexican Fish Salad

PREPARATION TIME About 20 minutes • **BAKING TIME** About 12 minutes • **CHILLING TIME** At least 2 hours

2 pounds (905 g) mahi mahi or
rockfish fillets

4 large tomatoes (about 2 lbs./
905 g total), coarsely diced

⅔ cup (160 ml) lime juice

3 cloves garlic, minced or pressed

1 cup (130 g) sliced pimento-stuffed
green olives

⅓ cup (40 g) drained capers

½ cup (50 g) thinly sliced green onions

Salt and pepper

About 12 large iceberg lettuce leaves
(about 6 oz./170 g total)

Lime wedges

Keep this chilled salad in mind for a summer lunch or dinner. Tomatoes, olives, and capers are tossed with lime juice and chunks of mahi mahi for a refreshing meal.

1 Rinse fish and pat dry. Place fish in a 9- by 13-inch (23- by 33-cm) baking dish, overlapping fillets slightly. Cover and bake in a 400°F (205°C) oven until opaque but still moist in thickest part; cut to test (about 12 minutes). Let cool; then cover and refrigerate for at least 2 hours or up to 1 day.

2 Lift fish from pan; discard pan juices. Pull out and discard any bones. Break fish into bite-size chunks. In a large bowl, combine fish, tomatoes, lime juice, garlic, olives, capers, and onions; mix gently. Season to taste with salt and pepper.

3 To serve, line a serving bowl with lettuce leaves; spoon in salad. Garnish with lime wedges.

PER SERVING

EXCHANGES
0 starch, 0 fruit, 0 milk,
0 other carbohydrates/sugar, 1½ vegetables,
3 very lean meat/protein, ½ fat

NUTRIENTS
152 calories (20% calories from fat), 3 g total fat,
0.5 g saturated fat, 83 mg cholesterol,
670 mg sodium, 8 g carbohydrates, 2 g fiber,
23 g protein, 40 mg calcium, 3 mg iron

MAKES 8 SERVINGS

Chicken Salad in Cantaloupe Halves

PREPARATION TIME About 25 minutes

These individual salads are perfect for a warm-weather brunch or lunch. You might complete the meal with warm bran muffins and iced tea.

1 In a large bowl, combine bell pepper, papaya, chicken, cilantro, and capers. (At this point, you may cover and refrigerate for up to 4 hours.)

2 In a small bowl, stir together lime peel, lime juice, and orange juice. Pour juice mixture over chicken mixture; stir to combine. Season to taste with salt and pepper.

3 To serve, cut each melon in half, then scoop out and discard seeds. If necessary, trim a thin slice from the base of each melon half so it sits steadily. Spoon chicken salad into melon halves; garnish with lime wedges.

1 medium-size yellow bell pepper
(about 6 oz./170 g), seeded and finely chopped

1 medium-size firm-ripe papaya
(about 1 lb./455 g), peeled, seeded, and cut into ½-inch (1-cm) cubes

3 cups (420 g) shredded cooked chicken

¼ cup (10 g) minced cilantro

2 tablespoons drained capers

2 teaspoons grated lime peel

¼ cup (60 ml) lime juice

¼ cup (60 ml) orange juice

Salt and pepper

2 small cantaloupes
(about 2¼ lbs./1.02 kg each)

Lime wedges

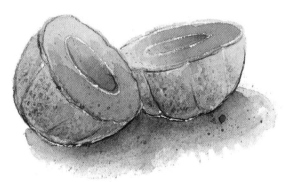

P E R   S E R V I N G

E X C H A N G E S
0 starch, 2 fruit, 0 milk,
0 other carbohydrates/sugar, ½ vegetable,
4 very lean meat/protein, 1½ fat

N U T R I E N T S
339 calories (23% calories from fat), 9 g total fat,
2 g saturated fat, 94 mg cholesterol,
229 mg sodium, 34 g carbohydrates, 3 g fiber,
34 g protein, 71 mg calcium, 2 mg iron

M A K E S   4   S E R V I N G S

Steak & Couscous with Raspberries

1 pound (455 g) lean boneless top sirloin steak (about 1 inch/2.5 cm thick), trimmed of fat

½ cup (120 ml) dry red wine

5 tablespoons (75 ml) raspberry vinegar or red wine vinegar

¼ cup (25 g) chopped green onions

2 tablespoons (30 ml) reduced-sodium soy sauce

1 tablespoon sugar

2 teaspoons chopped fresh tarragon or ½ teaspoon dried tarragon

1 tablespoon (18 g) raspberry or apple jelly

¾ cup (180 ml) fat-free reduced-sodium chicken broth

⅔ cup (160 ml) low-fat milk

¼ teaspoon ground coriander

6½ ounces/185 g (about 1 cup) dried couscous

1 tablespoon (15 ml) olive oil

8 cups (440 g) bite-size pieces red leaf lettuce leaves

2 cups (245 g) raspberries

Tarragon sprigs (optional)

When raspberries are in season, enjoy this quickly cooked beef and couscous salad. Fresh raspberries adorn the salad, and raspberry vinegar infuses the entire dish. Don't wash the raspberries until just before using them.

1 Slice steak across grain into strips about ⅛ inch (3 mm) thick and 3 inches (8 cm) long. Place meat, wine, 1 tablespoon (15 ml) of the vinegar, 2 tablespoons of the onions, soy sauce, 2 teaspoons of the sugar, and chopped tarragon in a large heavy-duty resealable plastic bag or large nonmetal bowl. Seal bag and rotate to coat meat (or stir meat in bowl and cover airtight). Refrigerate for at least 30 minutes or up to a day, turning (or stirring) occasionally.

2 Cook jelly in a 2- to 3-quart (1.9- to 2.8-liter) pan over low heat, stirring, until melted. Add broth, milk, and coriander; increase heat to medium-high and bring to a gentle boil. Stir in couscous. Cover, remove from heat, and let stand until liquid is absorbed (about 5 minutes).

3 Transfer couscous mixture to a large nonmetal bowl; let cool briefly, fluffing occasionally with a fork. Cover and refrigerate until cool (at least 30 minutes) or for up to 2 hours, fluffing occasionally. Meanwhile, heat 1 teaspoon of the oil in a wide nonstick frying pan over medium-high heat. Add meat and its juices and cook, stirring, until browned and done to your liking; cut to test (3 to 5 minutes). Transfer to a large nonmetal bowl and let cool.

4 Combine remaining 2 teaspoons oil, remaining 4 tablespoons (60 ml) vinegar, and remaining 1 teaspoon sugar in a large nonmetal bowl. Mix until blended. Add lettuce and turn to coat. Arrange lettuce on individual plates. Stir remaining 2 tablespoons onions into couscous mixture. Spoon onto lettuce, top with meat, and sprinkle with raspberries. Garnish with tarragon sprigs, if desired.

PER SERVING

EXCHANGES
2¼ starch, ½ fruit, 0 milk,
¼ other carbohydrates/sugar, 2 vegetables,
3¼ lean meat/protein, 0 fat

NUTRIENTS
456 calories (20% calories from fat), 10 g total fat,
3 g saturated fat, 71 mg cholesterol,
273 mg sodium, 55 g carbohydrates, 5 g fiber,
34 g protein, 151 mg calcium, 5 mg iron

MAKES 4 SERVINGS

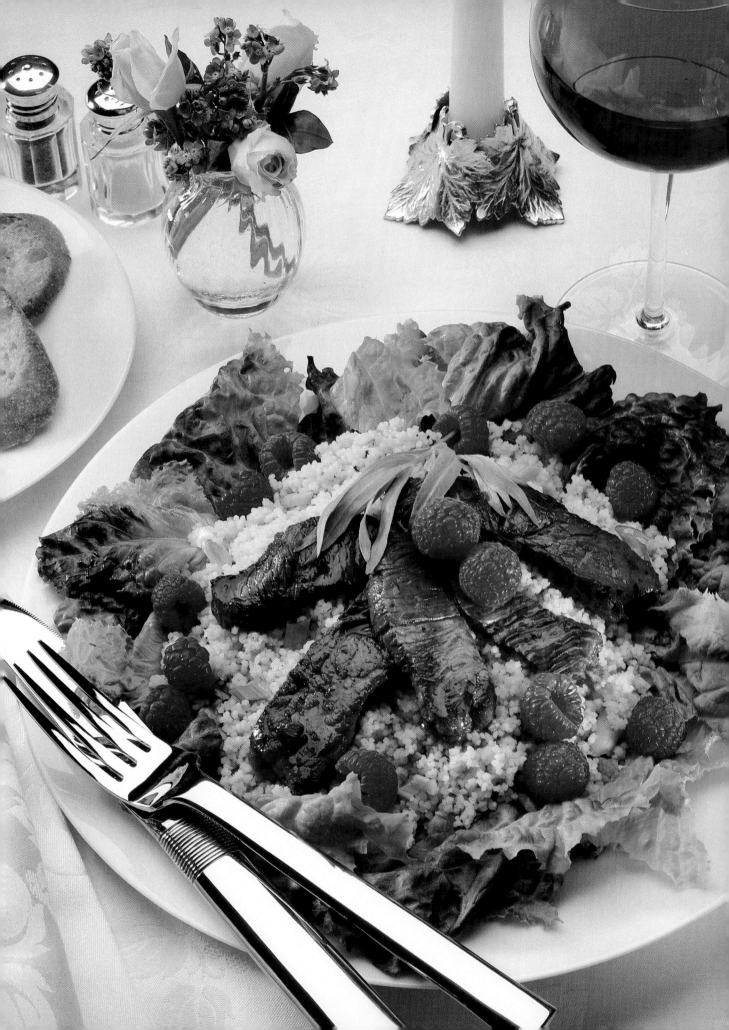

Cool Curry Turkey Salad

1 tablespoon (15 ml) olive oil

1 tablespoon minced fresh ginger

1 tablespoon curry powder

2 cups (280 g) diced cooked turkey or chicken

2½ cups (325 g) cold cooked rice

1 cup (240 ml) plain nonfat yogurt

¾ cup (75 g) thinly sliced green onions

½ cup (40 g) thinly sliced water chestnuts

¼ teaspoon salt

1 small honeydew melon (about 2½ lbs./1.15 kg)), seeded, cut into slender wedges, and peeled

Romaine lettuce leaves, rinsed and crisped

Lemon or lime wedges

Accompanied by slender wedges of honeydew melon, this piquant turkey-rice salad makes a tempting main dish for a warm evening.

1 Heat oil in a medium-size frying pan over medium heat. Add ginger and curry powder. Cook, stirring, just until seasonings are lightly browned (about 1 minute). Remove from heat and let cool slightly.

2 In a 2-quart (1.9 liter) bowl, combine ginger–curry powder mixture, turkey, rice, yogurt, ½ cup (50 g) of the onions, water chestnuts, and salt; mix lightly to blend. Cover and refrigerate for at least 1 hour or up to 3 hours.

3 Just before serving, arrange melon wedges on one side of a platter. Line other side of platter with lettuce leaves; mound turkey salad atop lettuce. Garnish with lemon or lime wedges and remaining ¼ cup (25 g) onions.

PER SERVING

EXCHANGES
1 starch, ½ fruit, ¼ skim milk, 0 other carbohydrates/sugar, 1 vegetable, 1½ very lean meat/protein, 1 fat

NUTRIENTS
247 calories (18% calories from fat), 5 g total fat, 1 g saturated fat, 37 mg cholesterol, 167 mg sodium, 32 g carbohydrates, 2 g fiber, 18 g protein, 115 mg calcium, 2 mg iron

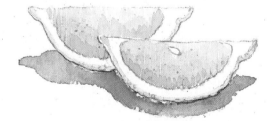

MAKES 6 SERVINGS

❖ Meats ❖

Hungarian Beef Stew

PREPARATION TIME About 20 minutes • **COOKING TIME** About 2 hours

Red bell pepper and a spoonful of paprika give this sturdy entrée its Hungarian character. When the stew is almost done, cook a package of eggless noodles to serve alongside.

1 In a wide 3½- to 4-quart (3.3- to 3.8-liter) pan, combine beef and ½ cup (120 ml) of the broth. Cover and cook over medium heat for 30 minutes. Uncover, add garlic and paprika, and continue to cook, stirring occasionally, until almost all liquid has evaporated and drippings are browned (about 30 minutes).

2 Meanwhile, trim and discard ends and all but 1½ inches (3.5 cm) of green tops from leeks; remove tough outer leaves. Split leeks lengthwise; rinse well, then cut crosswise into 1-inch (2.5-cm) lengths. Set aside.

3 Blend remaining 1¼ cups (300 ml) broth into stew, stirring to scrape browned bits free. Mix in leeks, bell pepper, mushrooms, salt, and pepper. Bring to a boil; reduce heat, cover, and simmer until beef is very tender when pierced (about 1 hour).

4 When beef is done, stir port and yogurt mixture into stew. Increase heat to medium-high and bring to a boil; then boil, stirring, until sauce is bubbly and thickened.

1½ pounds (680 g) boneless beef top round, trimmed of fat and cut into 1-inch (2.5-cm) cubes

1 can (about 14½ oz./415 g) beef broth

1 clove garlic, minced or pressed

1 tablespoon sweet Hungarian paprika

3 medium-size leeks (1 to 1½ lbs./455 to 680 g total)

1 large red bell pepper (about 8 oz./230 g), seeded and cut into 1-inch (2.5-cm) squares

8 ounces (230 g) small mushrooms

½ teaspoon salt

¼ teaspoon pepper

2 tablespoons (30 ml) port or Madeira

½ cup (120 ml) plain low-fat yogurt blended with 1 tablespoon cornstarch

P E R   S E R V I N G

E X C H A N G E S
0 starch, 0 fruit, 0 milk,
¼ other carbohydrates/sugar, 1¾ vegetables,
3½ very lean meat/protein, 1 fat

N U T R I E N T S
222 calories (20% calories from fat), 5 g total fat,
2 g saturated fat, 66 mg cholesterol,
505 mg sodium, 14 g carbohydrates, 2 g fiber,
29 g protein, 72 mg calcium, 4 mg iron

M A K E S   6   S E R V I N G S

Beef Skewers with Saffron Couscous

1½ pounds (680 g) lean boneless top sirloin steak (about 1 inch/2.5 cm thick), trimmed of fat

½ cup (120 ml) reduced-sodium soy sauce

2 tablespoons (30 ml) honey

2 tablespoons (30 ml) red wine vinegar

1 clove garlic, minced or pressed

½ teaspoon ground ginger

¼ teaspoon pepper

1 teaspoon olive oil

1 large onion (about 8 oz./230 g), chopped

2 cups (470 ml) nonfat milk

¾ cup (180 ml) fat-free reduced-sodium chicken broth

Large pinch of saffron threads or ⅛ teaspoon saffron powder, or to taste

10 ounces/285 g (about 1⅔ cups) dried couscous

¼ cup (20 g) freshly grated Parmesan cheese, or to taste

Tomato wedges

Italian parsley sprigs

M arinated beef kebabs rest on a fluffy bed of couscous tinged golden with saffron. This precious spice, harvested from a species of crocus, is often used in Spanish, Italian, and Indian cuisines. Buy saffron threads, if possible, since they keep their flavor longer than powdered saffron. Crush saffron threads just before using.

1 Slice steak across grain into strips about ¼ inch (6 mm) thick and 4 inches (10 cm) long (for easier slicing, freeze steak for about 30 minutes before cutting). Place meat, soy sauce, honey, vinegar, garlic, ginger, pepper, and 2 tablespoons (30 ml) water in a large heavy-duty resealable plastic bag or large nonmetal bowl. Seal bag and rotate to coat meat (or turn meat in bowl and cover airtight). Refrigerate for at least 30 minutes or up to a day, turning (or stirring) occasionally. Meanwhile, soak 12 wooden skewers (8 to 10 inches/20 to 25 cm long) in hot water to cover for at least 30 minutes.

2 Lift meat from marinade and drain, reserving marinade. Weave 2 or 3 meat slices on each skewer so meat lies flat. Place in a lightly oiled broiler pan without a rack and set aside.

3 Heat oil in a 2- to 3-quart (1.9- to 2.8-liter) pan over medium-high heat. Add onion and cook, stirring often, until soft (about 5 minutes). Add milk, broth, and saffron; bring just to a boil. Stir in couscous; cover, remove from heat, and let stand until liquid is absorbed (about 5 minutes).

4 Meanwhile, broil meat 3 to 4 inches (8 to 10 cm) below heat, basting with reserved marinade and turning as needed, until done to your liking; cut to test (about 5 minutes for medium-rare).

5 Fluff couscous with fork, adding cheese. Spoon onto platter and top with meat. Garnish with tomatoes and parsley. Offer guests 2 skewers each.

PER SERVING

EXCHANGES

2¾ starch, 0 fruit, 0 milk, ¼ other carbohydrates/sugar, ½ vegetable, 4 very lean meat/protein, 1¾ fat

NUTRIENTS

436 calories (18% calories from fat), 9 g total fat, 3 g saturated fat, 80 mg cholesterol, 1,334 mg sodium, 49 g carbohydrates, 2 g fiber, 38 g protein, 179 mg calcium, 4 mg iron

MAKES 6 SERVINGS

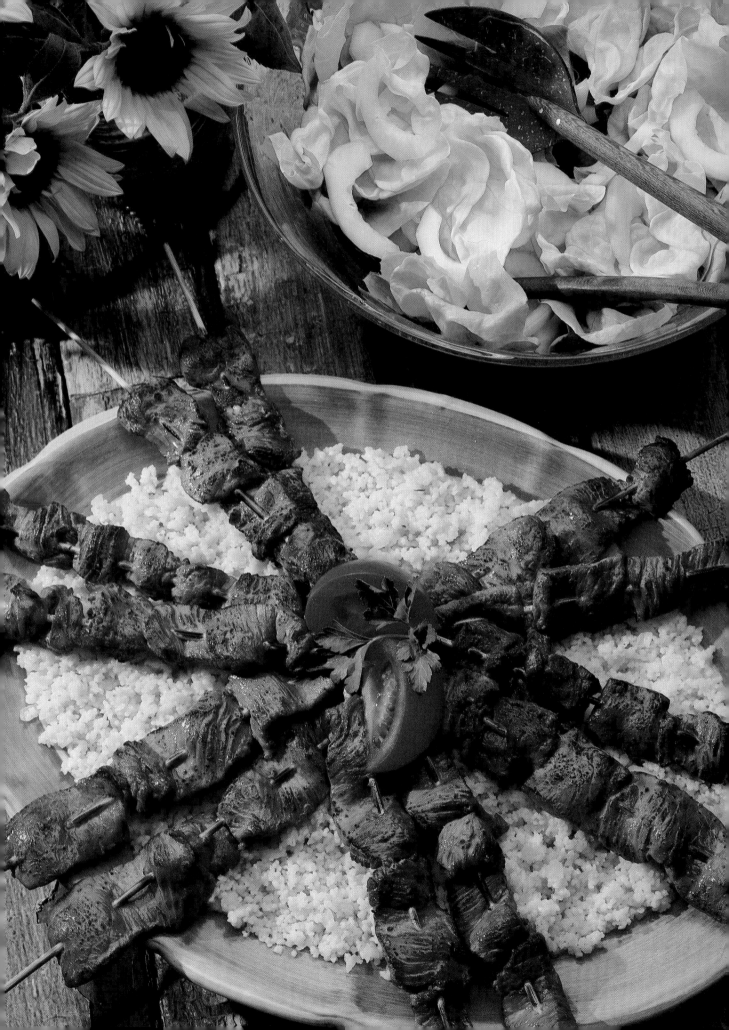

Low-Fat Spaghetti & Meatballs

PREPARATION TIME About 20 minutes • STANDING TIME About 15 minutes
BAKING TIME 25 to 30 minutes • COOKING TIME 35 to 40 minutes

¾ cup (132 g) bulgur

1½ cups (360 ml) boiling water

12 ounces (340 g) boneless beef top round, trimmed of fat (or use ground beef with 15 percent or less fat)

1 large onion (8 oz./230 g), chopped

4 cloves garlic, minced or pressed

1 teaspoon dried oregano

¼ teaspoon black pepper

About ½ teaspoon salt

4 ounces (115 g) mushrooms, sliced

1 tablespoon dried basil

¼ teaspoon crushed red pepper flakes

1 to 1¼ cups (240 to 300 ml) beef broth

1 large can (about 28 oz./795 g) crushed tomatoes

1 pound (455 g) dried spaghetti

Chopped parsley

Grated Parmesan cheese

An all-time family favorite, spaghetti and meatballs is one dish that's easily streamlined. We trimmed down the recipe by using a fat-free tomato-mushroom sauce and making the meatballs from very lean beef mixed with soaked bulgur; oven-browning the meatballs is another fat-sparing step. Because these meatballs soak up liquid readily, heat them only briefly in the sauce before serving.

1 In a large bowl, mix bulgur and boiling water. Let stand until bulgur is tender to bite (about 15 minutes).

2 Cut beef into ½-inch (1-cm) cubes and whirl in a food processor until coarsely ground (or put through a food chopper). In another large bowl, mix beef, onion, half the garlic, oregano, black pepper, and ½ teaspoon of the salt. Shape into ¼-cup (57-g) balls; place meatballs slightly apart in a lightly oiled shallow baking pan and bake in a 425°F (220°C) oven until well browned (25 to 30 minutes).

3 Meanwhile, in 5- to 6-quart (5- to 6-liter) pan, combine mushrooms, remaining garlic, basil, red pepper flakes, and ¼ cup (60 ml) water. Cook over high heat, stirring often, until liquid evaporates and vegetables begin to brown (about 10 minutes). To deglaze, add ¼ cup (60 ml) broth and stir to scrape browned bits free. Then continue to cook, stirring occasionally, until mixture begins to brown again. Repeat deglazing and browning steps one or two more times, using ¼ cup (60 ml) broth each time; mushrooms should be browned. Stir in tomatoes; reduce heat, cover, and simmer for 10 minutes. Add meatballs; cover and simmer for about 5 minutes. (Meatballs absorb liquid quickly; if sauce sticks, stir in a little broth.) Season to taste with salt.

4 While sauce is simmering, cook spaghetti in a 6- to 8-quart (6- to 8-liter) pan in about 4 quarts (3.8 liters) boiling water until just tender to bite (8 to 10 minutes); or cook according to package directions. Drain well. In pasta pan, bring ⅓ cup (80 ml) of the broth to a boil; return pasta to pan, stir to mix, and pour into a wide bowl.

5 To serve, top pasta with the meatballs and sprinkle with parsley. Offer cheese to add to taste.

PER SERVING

EXCHANGES
5¼ starch, 0 fruit, 0 milk,
0 other carbohydrates/sugar, 3½ vegetables,
1½ lean meat/protein, 0 fat

NUTRIENTS
562 calories (8% calories from fat), 5 g total fat,
1 g saturated fat, 39 mg cholesterol,
731 mg sodium, 97 g carbohydrates, 8 g fiber,
33 g protein, 107 mg calcium, 7 mg iron

MAKES 5 SERVINGS

Spinach Meat Loaf

PREPARATION TIME About 40 minutes • **BAKING TIME** About 1½ hours

Combining lean beef with ground turkey breast and grated potato helps cut the fat in this spinach-swirled, tomato-glazed meat loaf.

1 In a large nonmetal bowl, combine egg white, milk, and ½ cup (120 ml) of the tomato sauce; beat until well combined. Stir in bread crumbs, onion, potato, garlic, mustard, oregano, and pepper. Add beef and turkey; mix lightly. On a large sheet of plastic wrap, pat meat mixture into a 12-inch (30-cm) square. Distribute spinach over meat to within ½ inch (1 cm) of edges; sprinkle evenly with cheese.

2 Using plastic wrap to lift meat, roll up meat jelly roll style. Pinch seam and ends closed to seal in filling. Carefully place meat loaf, seam side down, in a shallow baking pan.

3 Bake meat loaf in a 350°F (175°C) oven for 1¼ hours. Meanwhile, in a small bowl, stir together sugar, vinegar, Worcestershire, and remaining tomato sauce until well blended. Set aside.

4 Remove pan from oven; spoon out and discard any drippings. Spoon tomato sauce mixture over meat loaf. Return to oven and continue to bake until meat is well browned (15 to 20 more minutes). With wide spatulas, carefully transfer meat loaf to a platter. Let stand for about 5 minutes before slicing.

1 large egg white

¼ cup (60 ml) evaporated skim milk

1 can (about 8 oz./230 g) tomato sauce

1½ cups (68 g) soft French bread crumbs

1 small onion (about 4 oz./115 g), finely chopped

1 large potato (about 8 oz./230 g), scrubbed and grated

1 clove garlic, minced or pressed

2 teaspoons Dijon mustard

¾ teaspoon dried oregano

¼ teaspoon pepper

1 pound (455 g) extra-lean ground beef

1 pound (455 g) ground skinless turkey breast

1 package (about 10 oz./285 g) frozen chopped spinach, thawed and squeezed dry

¼ cup (20 g) grated Romano or Parmesan cheese

1 tablespoon firmly packed brown sugar

1 tablespoon (15 ml) red wine vinegar

1¼ teaspoons Worcestershire

P E R   S E R V I N G

E X C H A N G E S
¾ starch, 0 fruit, 0 milk,
0 other carbohydrates/sugar, 1 vegetable,
3¼ lean meat/protein, 0 fat

N U T R I E N T S
258 calories (25% calories from fat), 7 g total fat,
2 g saturated fat, 73 mg cholesterol,
411 mg sodium, 18 g carbohydrates, 2 g fiber,
30 g protein, 115 mg calcium, 3 mg iron

M A K E S   8   S E R V I N G S

Penne all'Arrabbiata

PREPARATION TIME About 20 minutes • **COOKING TIME** 45 to 50 minutes

1 tablespoon (15 ml) olive oil

6 ounces (170 g) cooked ham, chopped

1 large onion (about 8 oz./230 g), finely chopped

½ cup (65 g) finely chopped carrot

½ cup (60 g) finely chopped celery

½ teaspoon crushed red pepper flakes

1 large can (about 28 oz./795 g) diced pear-shaped (Roma-type) tomatoes

1 pound (455 g) dried bite-size tube-shaped pasta such as penne or ziti

¼ cup (20 g) grated Parmesan cheese

Salt and black pepper

In Italy, *arrabbiata* means "angry"—and as the name suggests, this dish is fiery in flavor. Serve the spicy tomato sauce over quill-shaped pasta such as penne or ziti.

1 Heat oil in a 3- to 4-quart (2.8- to 3.8-liter) pan. Add ham and cook over medium-high heat, stirring often, until lightly browned (6 to 8 minutes). Add onion, carrot, celery, and red pepper flakes; reduce heat to medium and cook, stirring often, until vegetables are soft (about 15 minutes). Stir in tomatoes and bring to a boil; then reduce heat and simmer, uncovered, stirring often, until sauce is reduced to about 3½ cups /830 ml (25 to 30 minutes).

2 When sauce is almost done, cook pasta in a 6- to 8-quart (6- to 8-liter) pan in about 4 quarts (3.8 liters) boiling water until just tender to bite (10 to 12 minutes); or cook according to package directions. Drain well, pour into a large bowl, and keep warm.

3 To serve, mix sauce and cheese with pasta; season to taste with salt and black pepper.

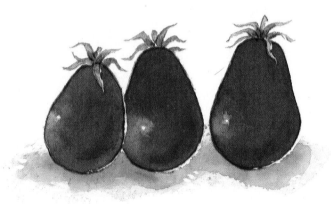

PER SERVING

EXCHANGES
4¼ starch, 0 fruit, 0 milk,
0 other carbohydrates/sugar, 2¼ vegetables,
1½ lean meat/protein, ¾ fat

NUTRIENTS
496 calories (16% calories from fat), 9 g total fat,
3 g saturated fat, 23 mg cholesterol,
866 mg sodium, 80 g carbohydrates, 5 g fiber,
23 g protein, 133 mg calcium, 5 mg iron

MAKES 5 SERVINGS

Cuban-Style Pork with Beans & Rice

PREPARATION TIME About 15 minutes • **MARINATING TIME** At least 4 hours
ROASTING TIME 35 to 55 minutes • **COOKING TIME** About 10 minutes

A compact roast leg of pork—sometimes called fresh ham—is marinated Caribbean style and served with rice and savory black beans.

1 Roll pork compactly, then tie securely with cotton string at 1½-inch (3.5-cm) intervals. Set a large heavy-duty plastic bag in a shallow pan. In bag, combine two-thirds of the garlic, oregano, cumin seeds, red pepper flakes, and lime juice; add pork. Seal bag and turn to coat pork with marinade; then refrigerate for at least 4 hours or up to 1 day, turning occasionally.

2 Lift pork from bag and drain briefly; reserve marinade. Place pork on a rack in a roasting pan and roast in a 350°F (175°C) oven, drizzling once or twice with marinade, until a meat thermometer inserted in thickest part registers 155°F/68°C (35 to 55 minutes). After 25 minutes, check temperature every 5 to 10 minutes.

3 Meanwhile, prepare black beans. Heat oil in a wide non-stick frying pan over medium heat. Add onion and bell pepper; cook, stirring often, until onion is soft but not browned (about 5 minutes). Stir in remaining garlic, ground cumin, and beans and their liquid. Cook, stirring, until heated through (about 3 minutes). Just before serving, stir in vinegar.

4 When pork is done, let it stand for about 5 minutes. Then thinly slice pork across the grain and transfer to a platter. Spoon rice alongside pork. Garnish pork and rice with green onions and lime wedges; serve with black beans.

1½ to 1¾ pounds (680 to 795 g) boneless fresh leg of pork, trimmed of fat

3 cloves garlic, minced or pressed

½ teaspoon dried oregano

¼ teaspoon cumin seeds, coarsely crushed

¼ teaspoon crushed red pepper flakes

¼ cup (60 ml) lime juice

2 teaspoons olive oil

1 medium-size onion (about 6 oz./170 g), thinly sliced

½ cup (75 g) finely chopped green bell pepper

½ teaspoon ground cumin

1 can (about 15 oz./425 g) black beans and their liquid (or use 2 cups/320 g drained cooked black beans, plus ⅓ cup/80 ml fat-free reduced-sodium chicken broth)

2 teaspoons cider vinegar

3 cups (390 g) hot cooked long-grain white rice

¼ cup (25 g) thinly sliced green onions

Lime wedges

P E R   S E R V I N G

E X C H A N G E S
2½ starch, 0 fruit, 0 milk,
0 other carbohydrates/sugar, 2 vegetables,
3¼ lean meat/protein, ½ fat

N U T R I E N T S
425 calories (27% calories from fat), 13 g
total fat, 4 g saturated fat, 88 mg cholesterol,
284 mg sodium, 43 g carbohydrates, 5 g fiber,
34 g protein, 57 mg calcium, 4 mg iron

M A K E S   6   S E R V I N G S

Pork Tenderloin with Peanut Vermicelli

PREPARATION TIME About 20 minutes • **COOKING TIME** About 35 minutes

2 pork tenderloins (about 12 oz./340 g each), trimmed of fat and membrane

¼ cup (60 ml) hoisin sauce

3 tablespoons firmly packed brown sugar

2 tablespoons (30 ml) dry sherry

2 tablespoons (30 ml) reduced-sodium soy sauce

1 tablespoon (15 ml) lemon juice

12 ounces (340 g) dried vermicelli

½ cup (160 g) plum butter or plum jam

¼ cup (60 ml) seasoned rice vinegar (or ¼ cup/60 ml distilled white vinegar and 2 teaspoons sugar)

¼ cup (65 g) creamy peanut butter

3 tablespoons (45 ml) Oriental sesame oil

2 cloves garlic, minced or pressed

⅛ teaspoon ground ginger

¼ teaspoon crushed red pepper flakes

1 package (about 10 oz./285 g) frozen tiny peas, thawed

⅓ cup (15 g) cilantro

Sliced kumquats (optional)

2 tablespoons chopped peanuts (optional)

P E R   S E R V I N G

E X C H A N G E S
3 starch, 0 fruit, 0 milk,
2½ other carbohydrates/sugar, 0 vegetables,
4 lean meat/protein, 1 fat

N U T R I E N T S
646 calories (25% calories from fat), 18 g
total fat, 3 g saturated fat, 67 mg cholesterol,
788 mg sodium, 83 g carbohydrates, 4 g fiber,
37 g protein, 43 mg calcium, 5 mg iron

Peanuts, plum butter (a condiment like apple butter), and sweet and spicy hoisin sauce enhance this roast pork dish. Hoisin sauce—a mixture of soybeans, garlic, chile peppers, and spices—is available in bottles and cans at Asian markets and many large supermarkets.

1 Place tenderloins on a rack in a 9- by 13-inch (23- by 33-cm) baking pan. In a bowl, stir together hoisin, brown sugar, sherry, 1 tablespoon (15 ml) of the soy sauce, and lemon juice. Brush over pork, reserving remaining mixture.

2 Roast pork in a 450°F (230°C) oven, brushing with remaining marinade, until a meat thermometer inserted in thickest part registers 155°F/68°C (20 to 30 minutes; after 15 minutes, check temperature every 5 minutes). If drippings begin to burn, add 4 to 6 tablespoons (60 to 90 ml) water, stirring to loosen browned bits.

3 Meanwhile, bring 12 cups (2.8 liters) water to a boil in a 5- to 6-quart (5- to 6-liter) pan over medium-high heat. Stir in pasta and cook just until tender to bite (8 to 10 minutes); or cook according to package directions. Drain well and keep warm.

4 Transfer meat to a board, cover loosely, and let stand for 10 minutes. Skim and discard fat from pan drippings. Pour drippings and any juices on board into a small serving container; keep warm.

5 Meanwhile, combine plum butter, vinegar, peanut butter, oil, garlic, ginger, red pepper flakes, and remaining 1 tablespoon (15 ml) soy sauce in 5- to 6-quart (5- to 6-liter) pan. Bring to a boil over medium heat and cook, whisking, just until smooth. Remove from heat and add pasta, peas, and cilantro. Lift with 2 forks to mix. Mound pasta on individual plates. Thinly slice meat across grain; arrange on pasta. Garnish with kumquats, if desired. Offer juices and, if desired, peanuts to add to taste.

M A K E S   6   S E R V I N G S

Pork Tenderloin with Peanut Vermicelli ▶

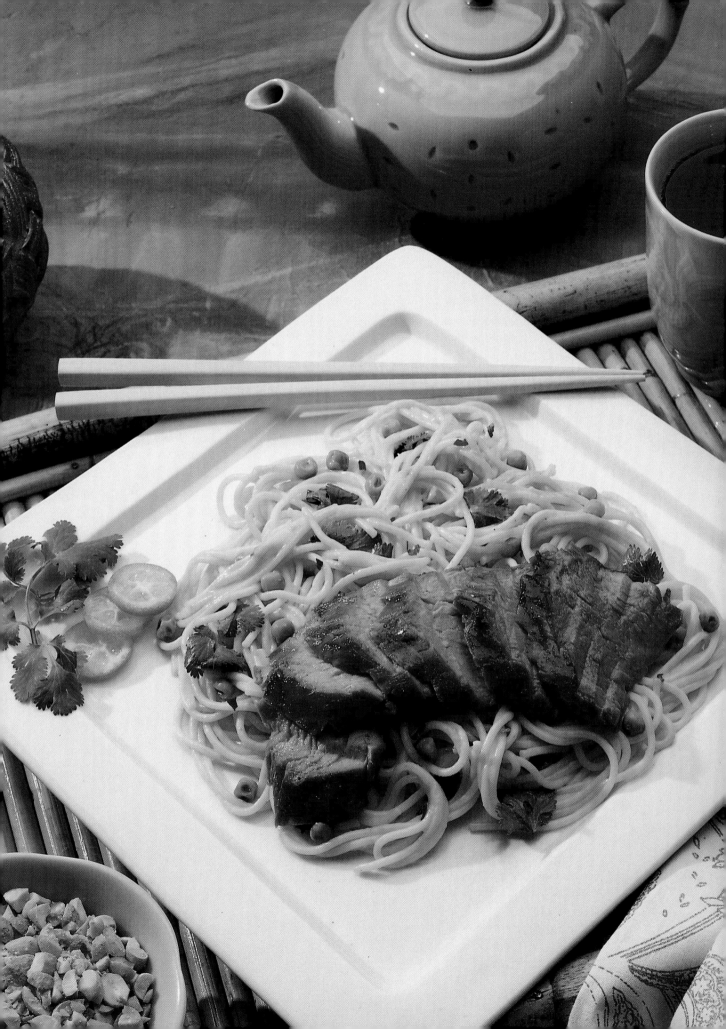

Garlic Pork Chops with Balsamic Vinegar

PREPARATION TIME 15 to 20 minutes • **COOKING TIME** About 20 minutes

1 small head garlic (about 1½ oz./45 g),
separated into cloves

6 center-cut loin pork chops
(about 2 lbs./905 g total),
trimmed of fat

Pepper

Vegetable oil cooking spray

12 ounces (340 g) dried medium-wide
eggless noodles

¼ cup (60 ml) sweet vermouth

1 tablespoon (15 ml) Dijon mustard

⅓ cup (80 ml) balsamic vinegar

Salt

Chopped parsley

Dark, rich-tasting balsamic vinegar is a specialty from the area around Modena, Italy. Combined with mustard and vermouth, it makes a tempting sauce for juicy pork chops sautéed with plenty of garlic.

1 In a medium-size pan, bring about 4 cups (950 ml) water to a boil. Add unpeeled garlic cloves and boil for 1 minute; drain. Let garlic cool slightly, then peel cloves and set aside.

2 Sprinkle pork chops generously with pepper. Coat a wide frying pan with cooking spray and place over medium-high heat. Add chops and cook until well browned on bottom (4 to 5 minutes); turn chops over, arrange garlic cloves around them, and continue to cook until chops are browned on other side (4 to 5 more minutes).

3 Meanwhile, in a 5- to 6-quart (5- to 6-liter) pan, cook noodles in about 3 quarts (2.8 liters) boiling water until just tender to bite (7 to 9 minutes); or cook according to package directions. Drain well, pour onto a deep platter, and keep warm.

4 While noodles are cooking, in a small cup, mix vermouth and mustard; pour over browned chops. Reduce heat to low, cover, and cook until chops are done but still moist and slightly pink in center; cut to test (about 5 minutes). Arrange chops over noodles and keep warm.

5 Add vinegar to sauce in pan. Increase heat to medium-high and stir to scrape browned bits free. Bring to a boil; then boil, uncovered, until sauce is reduced to about ½ cup/120 ml (2 to 3 minutes). Season to taste with salt. Spoon sauce over chops; sprinkle chops and noodles with parsley.

PER SERVING

EXCHANGES
2¾ starch, 0 fruit, 0 milk,
0 other carbohydrates/sugar, 1 vegetable,
3¼ very-lean meat/protein, 1¼ fat

NUTRIENTS
366 calories (21% calories from fat), 6 g total fat,
2 g saturated fat, 62 mg cholesterol,
140 mg sodium, 43 g carbohydrates, 2 g fiber,
30 g protein, 45 mg calcium, 3 mg iron

MAKES 6 SERVINGS

Lentil Cassoulet

Traditional *cassoulet* is made with white beans, but we've substituted lentils to cut down on cooking time. Thick with sausage and meaty pork ribs, the hearty dish is an excellent choice for entertaining: It serves a crowd, and it can be assembled—all ready to slip into the oven for final baking—up to a day ahead of time.

1 Cut pork ribs apart between bones. Mix salt, sugar, and pepper; rub all over pork. Place pork in a large heavy-duty plastic bag; seal bag and refrigerate for at least 6 hours or up to 1 day, turning occasionally. Rinse pork well and pat dry.

2 Place pork and whole sausage in a single layer in a 10- by 15-inch (25 - by 38-cm) rimmed baking pan; bake in a 450°F (230°C) oven until browned (about 30 minutes). Discard fat from pan; set ribs and sausage aside.

3 In a 6- to 8-quart (6- to 8-liter) pan, combine 1 cup (240 ml) of the broth, onions, garlic, thyme, coriander seeds, and bay leaf. Cook over high heat, stirring often, until liquid evaporates and onions begin to brown (about 10 minutes). To deglaze, add ⅓ cup (80 ml) more broth and stir to scrape browned bits free. Then continue to cook, stirring occasionally, until mixture begins to brown again. Repeat deglazing and browning steps 1 or 2 more times, using ⅓ cup (80 ml) broth each time; onions should be well browned.

4 Add lentils, pork ribs, 8 cups (1.9 liters) of the broth, and carrots to pan. Bring to a boil; then reduce heat, cover, and simmer until lentils are tender to bite (30 to 40 minutes). Meanwhile, cut sausage into ¼-inch-thick (6-mm-thick) diagonal slices.

5 With a slotted spoon, lift pork ribs from lentil mixture and set aside; then pour lentil mixture into a shallow 5- to 6-quart (5- to 6-liter) casserole (about 12 by 16 inches/30 by 40 cm). Nestle sausage slices and ribs into lentils. Cover casserole tightly. (At this point, you may let cool, then refrigerate for up to 1 day.)

6 Bake, covered, in a 350°F (175°C) oven until hot in center (about 35 minutes; about 1½ hours if refrigerated). Mix bread crumbs and oil; uncover casserole and sprinkle with crumbs. Continue to bake, uncovered, until crumbs are golden (20 to 25 more minutes). Sprinkle with parsley.

3 to 4 pounds (1.35 to 1.8 kg) country-style pork ribs, trimmed of fat

2 tablespoons salt

2 tablespoons sugar

1 teaspoon pepper

1 pound (455 g) turkey kielbasa

About 10 cups (2.4 liters) fat-free reduced-sodium chicken broth

2 large onions (about 1 lb./455 g total), chopped

3 cloves garlic, minced or pressed

2 teaspoons dried thyme

2 teaspoons coriander seeds

1 dried bay leaf

2 pounds (905 g) lentils, rinsed and drained

3 large carrots (about 10½ oz./300 g total), coarsely chopped

1 cup (45 g) coarse soft bread crumbs

2 teaspoons olive oil

2 tablespoons chopped parsley

P E R   S E R V I N G

E X C H A N G E S
4.5 starch, 0 fruit, 0 milk,
0 other carbohydrates/sugar, 1 vegetable,
5 lean meat/protein, 0 fat

N U T R I E N T S
620 calories (21% calories from fat), 15 g total fat, 6 g saturated fat, 75 mg cholesterol, 1,174 mg sodium, 73 g carbohydrates, 14 g fiber, 56 g protein, 125 mg calcium, 11 mg iron

M A K E S   9   S E R V I N G S

Orange Lamb Chops with Hominy

6 tablespoons (90 ml) orange juice

About 5 tablespoons (75 ml) lime juice

⅛ to ¼ teaspoon sugar

1 clove garlic, minced or pressed

1 teaspoon minced shallot

Salt and pepper

8 lamb rib chops (about 2 lbs./905 g total), cut 1 inch (2.5 cm) thick

3 cans (about 14 oz./400 g each) yellow hominy, drained

1 teaspoon olive oil or vegetable oil

2 teaspoons water

1 tablespoon chopped fresh oregano or 1 teaspoon dried oregano

3 tablespoons finely chopped parsley

The tart-sweet orange-juice mixture that flavors these lamb chops is a popular dressing and marinade on the Yucatán peninsula. The authentic recipe calls for sour Seville oranges, but you can use regular orange juice, too; just be sure to sharpen the flavor with lime (as we do here). And to give the dressing its special zing, don't forget to add a light sprinkling of salt just before serving.

1 In a nonmetal bowl, mix orange juice, lime juice (enough to give orange juice a tart flavor), sugar, garlic, shallot, and about ⅛ teaspoon pepper.

2 Trim and discard fat from lamb chops. Place chops in a large (1-gallon/3.8-liter) heavy-duty resealable plastic bag or large nonmetal bowl. Pour ¼ cup (60 ml) of the orange dressing over chops; reserve remaining dressing. Seal bag and rotate to coat chops (or turn chops in bowl to coat, then cover airtight). Refrigerate for at least 30 minutes or until next day, turning occasionally.

3 To prepare hominy, in a wide nonstick frying pan, combine hominy, oil, water, and oregano. Cook over medium-high heat, stirring, until hominy is hot (about 5 minutes). Season to taste with salt and pepper and keep warm.

4 Lift chops from marinade and drain; discard marinade. Place chops on lightly oiled rack of a broiler pan. Broil chops about 6 inches (15 cm) below heat, turning once, until done to your liking; cut to test (8 to 10 minutes for medium-rare).

5 Transfer chops to dinner plates or a platter; spoon hominy alongside chops. Sprinkle with parsley. Offer remaining orange dressing and salt to add to taste.

PER SERVING

EXCHANGES
4 starch, 0 fruit, 0 milk,
0 other carbohydrates/sugar, 0 vegetables,
2 lean meat/protein, 1½ fat

NUTRIENTS
425 calories (29% calories from fat), 13 g
total fat, 4 g saturated fat, 66 mg cholesterol,
735 mg sodium, 49 g carbohydrates, 8 g fiber,
25 g protein, 56 mg calcium, 4 mg iron

MAKES 4 SERVINGS

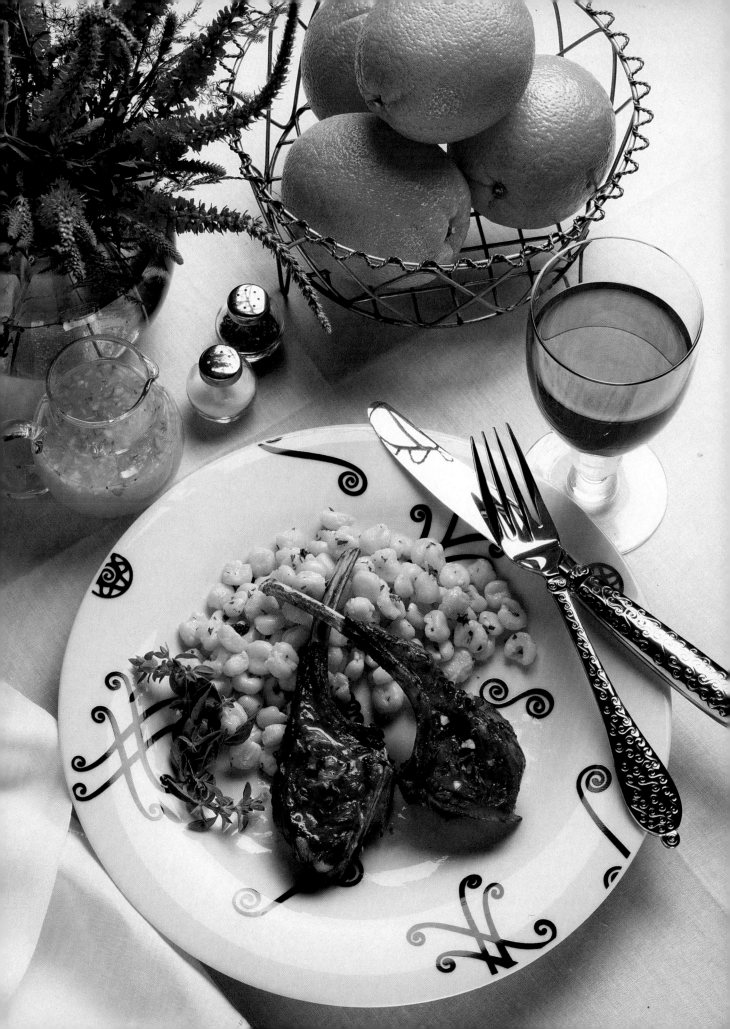

Cider-Baked Lamb Stew with Turnips

3 tablespoons all-purpose flour

½ teaspoon ground cloves

¼ teaspoon ground white pepper

2 pounds (905 g) boneless leg of lamb, trimmed of fat and cut into 1-inch (2.5-cm) cubes

1½ cups (360 ml) apple cider

4 medium-size turnips (about 1¼ lbs./565 g total), peeled and cut lengthwise into wedges

2 medium-size onions (about 12 oz./340 g total), sliced

1 clove garlic, minced or pressed

⅓ cup (20 g) chopped parsley

Salt

In this easy version of a French country favorite, floured lamb cubes are browned in a hot oven, then simmered in cider until tender. Complement the stew with baked sweet potatoes and steamed fresh spinach, if you like.

1 Combine flour, cloves, and white pepper. Coat lamb cubes with flour mixture and arrange slightly apart in an ungreased shallow 3- to 3½-quart (2.8- to 3.3-liter) baking dish. Bake in a 500°F (260°C) oven for 20 minutes, then remove from oven and let cool in baking dish for about 5 minutes.

2 Reduce oven temperature to 375°F (190°C). Gradually add cider to lamb in baking dish, stirring to scrape browned bits free. Add turnips, onions, garlic, and all but 1 tablespoon of the parsley.

3 Cover tightly and bake until lamb and turnips are very tender when pierced (1½ to 2 hours), stirring occasionally. Skim and discard fat from stew, if necessary. Season to taste with salt. Sprinkle with reserved 1 tablespoon parsley.

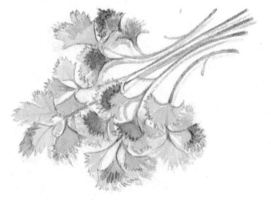

PER SERVING

EXCHANGES
¼ starch, ¼ fruit, 0 milk,
0 other carbohydrates/sugar, 1¼ vegetables,
3 very lean meat/protein, 1 fat

NUTRIENTS
211 calories (23% calories from fat), 5 g total fat,
2 g saturated fat, 73 mg cholesterol,
113 mg sodium, 15 g carbohydrates, 2 g fiber,
25 g protein, 41 mg calcium, 3 mg iron

MAKES 8 SERVINGS

Veal Stew with Caraway

PREPARATION TIME About 15 minutes • **COOKING TIME** About 1¾ hours

This delicate veal stew is at its best served over helpings of hot, tender noodles. Caraway seeds are typical of German and other northern European cuisines.

1 In a wide 3½- to 4-quart (3.3- to 3.8-liter) pan, combine veal, oil, salt, white pepper, onion, and wine. Cover and cook over medium-low heat for 30 minutes. Uncover pan and stir in caraway seeds. Increase heat to medium and continue to cook, stirring occasionally, until almost all liquid has evaporated and onion is browned (15 to 20 minutes). Add broth and carrots to pan, stirring to scrape browned bits free.

2 Reduce heat to low, cover, and simmer until veal is tender when pierced (35 to 45 minutes). Increase heat to medium and cook, uncovered, stirring often, until sauce is slightly thickened (12 to 15 minutes). To serve, spoon stew over noodles; sprinkle with parsley.

1 to 1½ pounds (455 to 680 g) boneless veal shoulder, trimmed of fat and cut into 1-inch (2.5-cm) cubes

1 tablespoon (15 ml) olive oil or vegetable oil

¼ teaspoon salt

⅛ teaspoon ground white pepper

1 large onion (about 8 oz./230 g), finely chopped

½ cup (120 ml) dry white wine

2 teaspoons caraway seeds

1 can (about 14½ oz./415 g) fat-free reduced-sodium chicken broth

2 medium-size carrots (about 5 oz./140 g total), chopped

3 to 4 cups (325 to 410 g) hot cooked eggless noodles

Chopped parsley

PER SERVING

EXCHANGES
1¼ starch, 0 fruit, 0 milk,
0 other carbohydrates/sugar, 1¼ vegetables,
3 very lean meat/protein, 1½ fat

NUTRIENTS
286 calories (24% calories from fat), 8 g total fat,
2 g saturated fat, 98 mg cholesterol,
270 mg sodium, 27 g carbohydrates, 3 g fiber,
28 g protein, 62 mg calcium, 2 mg iron

MAKES 5 SERVINGS

Baked Polenta with Veal Sauce

PREPARATION TIME About 15 minutes • **BAKING TIME** 40 to 45 minutes • **COOKING TIME** About 25 minutes

4 cups (950 ml) fat-free reduced-sodium chicken broth

1¼ cups (173 g) polenta

¾ cup (129 g) finely chopped onion

1 tablespoon (15 ml) plus 1 teaspoon olive oil

1 small carrot (about 2 oz./55 g), shredded

4 ounces (115 g) mushrooms, quartered

1 clove garlic, minced or pressed

2 teaspoons Italian herb seasoning (or ½ teaspoon each dried basil, dried marjoram, dried oregano, and dried thyme)

1 pound (455 g) lean ground veal

1 large can (about 28 oz./795 g) pear-shaped (Roma-style) tomatoes

¼ cup (65 g) tomato paste

½ cup (120 ml) dry white wine

Salt and pepper

Grated Parmesan cheese (optional)

S oft, creamy baked polenta is delicious on its own as a side dish—but even better when topped with a lean, herb-seasoned veal and tomato sauce.

1 To prepare polenta, in an oiled shallow 2-quart (1.9-liter) baking dish, mix broth, polenta, ¼ cup (43 g) of the onion, and 1 tablespoon (15 ml) of the olive oil. Bake in a 350°F (175°C) oven until all the liquid has been absorbed (40 to 45 minutes).

2 While polenta is baking, combine remaining 1 teaspoon oil, remaining ½ cup (86 g) onion, carrot, mushrooms, garlic, and herb seasoning in a wide nonstick frying pan. Cook over medium heat, stirring often, until onion is soft (about 5 minutes). Crumble veal into pan; cook, stirring often, until it begins to brown.

3 Cut up tomatoes; then add tomatoes and their liquid, tomato paste, and wine to pan. Bring to a boil. Adjust heat so sauce boils gently; cook, stirring occasionally, until thickened (about 20 minutes). Season to taste with salt and pepper.

4 Spoon polenta into wide, shallow bowls and top with veal sauce. Offer cheese to add to taste, if desired.

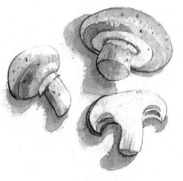

PER SERVING

EXCHANGES
1¾ starch, 0 fruit, 0 milk,
0 other carbohydrates/sugar, 2¾ vegetables,
2¼ very lean meat/protein, 2½ fat

NUTRIENTS
393 calories (30% calories from fat), 3 g total fat,
4 g saturated fat, 75 mg cholesterol,
543 mg sodium, 43 g carbohydrates, 5 g fiber,
26 g protein, 74 mg calcium, 4 mg iron

MAKES 5 SERVINGS

Turkey Curry with Soba

⟨▪◁◘▷▪◁◘▷▪◁◘▷▪◁◘▷▪◁◘▷▪◁◘▷▪◁◘▷▪◁◘▷▪◁◘▷▪◁◘▷▪◁◘▷▪◁◘▷▪◁◘▷▪◁◘▷▪◁◘▷▪◁◘▷▪◁◘▷▪◁◘⟩

PREPARATION TIME About 10 minutes • **COOKING TIME** About 40 minutes

To make this dish, you mix your own curry powder by blending a variety of spices. You'll be pleasantly surprised at the difference in taste when compared with store-bought curry powder. If you can't find *soba* noodles in the Asian foods section of your supermarket, substitute spaghettini.

1 Heat oil in a wide frying pan over medium heat. Add turkey and cook, stirring often, until browned on all sides (about 6 minutes). Using a slotted spoon, remove turkey from pan.

2 Add onion and garlic to pan; cook, stirring occasionally, until onion is soft (about 10 minutes). Add ginger, red pepper flakes, coriander, cumin, turmeric, and fennel seeds; cook, stirring, for 1 minute.

3 Return turkey to pan. Add broth and bring to a boil. Then reduce heat, cover, and simmer until meat is no longer pink in center (about 20 minutes); cut to test. Remove from heat.

4 While turkey is simmering, cook noodles in boiling water according to package directions until just tender to bite; drain well and pour into a large, shallow serving bowl.

5 Stir yogurt into turkey mixture, then pour mixture over noodles. Sprinkle with cashews.

1 tablespoon (15 ml) vegetable oil

1 pound (455 g) skinless, boneless turkey breast, cut into 1½-inch (3.5-cm) chunks

1 large onion (about 8 oz./230 g), thinly sliced

1 clove garlic, minced or pressed

1 tablespoon grated fresh ginger

1 teaspoon crushed red pepper flakes

1 teaspoon ground coriander

1 teaspoon ground cumin

1 teaspoon ground turmeric

½ teaspoon fennel seeds

1 cup (240 ml) fat-free reduced-sodium chicken broth

1 package (about 7 oz./200 g) dried soba noodles

1 cup (240 ml) plain nonfat yogurt

¼ cup (45 g) unsalted dry-roasted cashews

P E R   S E R V I N G

E X C H A N G E S
1¾ starch, ¼ fruit, 0 milk,
0 other carbohydrates/sugar, ½ vegetable,
2¾ very lean meat/protein, 1¼ fat

N U T R I E N T S
293 calories (19% calories from fat), 6 g total fat,
1 g saturated fat, 48 mg cholesterol,
350 mg sodium, 34 g carbohydrates, 2 g fiber,
28 g protein, 115 mg calcium, 3 mg iron

M A K E S   6   S E R V I N G S

Picadillo Stew

PREPARATION TIME About 15 minutes • **COOKING TIME** About 20 minutes

2 tablespoons slivered almonds

¼ cup (60 ml) dry red wine

2 tablespoons (30 ml) reduced-sodium soy sauce

1 tablespoon (15 ml) lemon juice

2 teaspoons sugar

1 teaspoon ground cumin

1 teaspoon ground coriander

1 teaspoon chili powder

⅛ teaspoon ground cinnamon

4 teaspoons cornstarch

1 teaspoon olive oil

1 pound (455 g) skinless, boneless turkey breast, cut into 1-inch (2.5-cm) chunks

1 large onion (about 8 oz./230 g), chopped

2 cloves garlic, minced or pressed

1 can (about 14½ oz./415 g) tomatoes

⅔ cup (100 g) raisins

Pepper

The recipe's name comes from the word *picar*, "to mince," so it's no surprise that the dish is made with chopped ingredients. This version is a hearty turkey stew, rich with raisins, spices, and almonds.

1 Toast almonds in a small frying pan over medium heat until golden (about 5 minutes), stirring often. Pour out of pan and set aside.

2 In a small nonmetal bowl, stir together wine, soy sauce, lemon juice, sugar, cumin, coriander, chili powder, cinnamon, and cornstarch. Set aside.

3 Heat oil in a wide nonstick frying pan or 6-quart (6-liter) pan over high heat. Add turkey, onion, and garlic. Cook, stirring, until onion is soft and meat is no longer pink in center; cut to test (10 to 15 minutes). If pan appears dry, add water, 1 tablespoon (15 ml) at a time. Cut up tomatoes; then add tomatoes and their liquid, wine mixture, and raisins to pan. Bring to a boil; then boil, stirring, just until thickened. Season to taste with pepper.

4 To serve, ladle stew into bowls and sprinkle with almonds.

PER SERVING

EXCHANGES
0 starch, 1¼ fruit, 0 milk,
½ other carbohydrates/sugar, 1¾ vegetables,
3½ very lean meat/protein, 1 fat

NUTRIENTS
317 calories (14% calories from fat), 5 g total fat,
0.7 g saturated fat, 70 mg cholesterol,
538 mg sodium, 36 g carbohydrates, 4 g fiber,
32 g protein, 87 mg calcium, 3 mg iron

MAKES 4 SERVINGS

Summer Turkey Stir-Fry

PREPARATION TIME About 15 minutes • **COOKING TIME** About 15 minutes

The secret to this vibrant stir-fry lies in the crisp fresh vegetables and the subtle sauce. You should have all the ingredients prepared before you begin cooking.

1 To prepare sauce, in a small bowl, mix broth, soy sauce, and cornstarch. Set aside.

2 In a 2- to 3-quart (1.9- to 2.8-liter) pan, bring 1½ cups (360 ml) of the water to a boil over high heat; stir in bulgur. Reduce heat, cover, and simmer until bulgur is tender to bite and water has been absorbed (about 15 minutes).

3 Meanwhile, heat oil in a wide frying pan or wok over high heat. Add garlic and turkey, and cook, stirring, until meat is no longer pink in center; cut to test (about 5 minutes). Add carrots, zucchini, ginger, and remaining ¼ cup (60 ml) water. Cover and continue to cook, stirring occasionally, until vegetables are tender-crisp to bite (about 5 more minutes). Uncover, bring to a boil, and boil until almost all liquid has evaporated. Stir in sauce; boil, stirring, until sauce is bubbly and thickened.

4 To serve, spoon bulgur onto individual plates and top with turkey mixture. Sprinkle with onions.

½ cup (120 ml) fat-free reduced-sodium chicken broth

2 tablespoons (30 ml) reduced-sodium soy sauce

1 tablespoon cornstarch

1¾ cups (420 ml) water

1 cup (175 g) bulgur

1 tablespoon (15 ml) vegetable oil or olive oil

3 cloves garlic, minced or pressed

1 pound (455 g) skinless, boneless turkey breast, cut into ¾-inch (2-cm) chunks

3 cups (390 g) thinly sliced carrots

2 small zucchini (about 8 oz./230 g total), sliced

2 tablespoons minced fresh ginger

½ cup (50 g) thinly sliced green onions

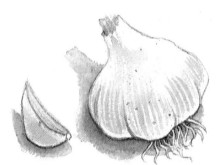

PER SERVING

EXCHANGES
2 starch, 0 fruit, 0 milk,
0 other carbohydrates/sugar, 2 vegetables,
3 very lean meat/protein, 1 fat

NUTRIENTS
344 calories (13% calories from fat), 5 g total fat,
0.9 g saturated fat, 70 mg cholesterol,
409 mg sodium, 41 g carbohydrates, 10 g fiber,
35 g protein, 72 mg calcium, 3 mg iron

MAKES 4 SERVINGS

Bean & Turkey Burritos

PREPARATION TIME About 40 minutes • **STANDING TIME** At least 1 hour • **COOKING TIME** About 2 hours

1 pound (455 g) dried red beans

2 medium-size onions (about 12 oz./340 g total), chopped

5 cups (1.2 liters) fat-free reduced-sodium chicken broth

½ cup (60 g) chili powder

½ cup (110 g) firmly packed brown sugar

2 whole star anise or 1 teaspoon anise seeds

4 cups (280 g) finely shredded red cabbage

1 cup (100 g) sliced green onions

⅓ cup (15 g) minced cilantro

¼ cup (60 ml) lime juice

½ teaspoon pepper

4 cups (560 g) bite-size pieces of cooked turkey

Salt

12 warm large flour tortillas (each 9 to 10 inches/23 to 25 cm in diameter)

Plain nonfat yogurt

Chili-seasoned red beans combined with leftover roast turkey make a superb filling for warm flour tortillas. Accompany the meal with a crisp, tart red cabbage salsa; it's good spooned into the burritos or simply offered alongside.

1 Rinse and sort beans, discarding any debris. Drain beans and place in a 6- to 8-quart (6- to 8-liter) pan; add 8 cups (1.9 liters) water. Bring to a boil over high heat; boil for 2 minutes. Then cover, remove from heat, and let stand for at least 1 hour. Drain beans, discarding water.

2 To pan, add onions, 5 cups (1.2 liters) water, broth, chili powder, sugar, and star anise; bring to a boil over high heat. Add beans to pan. Reduce heat, cover, and simmer gently until beans are very tender to bite (about 1½ hours). Drain beans, reserving cooking liquid. Discard star anise. (At this point, you may let beans and liquid cool, then cover separately and refrigerate for up to 2 days.)

3 To prepare red cabbage salsa, in a large bowl, combine cabbage, green onions, cilantro, lime juice, and pepper. Set aside.

4 Return cooking liquid to pan. Bring to a boil over high heat; then boil, uncovered, until reduced to about 3 cups (710 ml). Add beans and mash to make mixture as thick as you like. Add turkey and stir gently until mixture is hot. Season to taste with salt.

5 Spoon turkey mixture onto tortillas; add red cabbage salsa and yogurt to taste. Roll to enclose filling.

PER SERVING

EXCHANGES
3½ starch, 0 fruit, 0 milk,
½ other carbohydrates/sugar, 2 vegetables,
2 very lean meat/protein, 1¾ fat

NUTRIENTS
467 calories (16% calories from fat), 9 g total fat,
2 g saturated fat, 36 mg cholesterol,
410 mg sodium, 71 g carbohydrates, 9 g fiber,
30 g protein, 167 mg calcium, 6 mg iron

MAKES 12 SERVINGS

Apple Turkey Loaf

PREPARATION TIME About 25 minutes • **BAKING TIME** About 1 hour

Lightly blend spices and tart green apples with ground turkey breast for a lean, moist meat loaf. It's wonderful hot, and just as tasty served cold in sandwiches.

1 Melt butter in a wide frying pan over medium heat. Add apples and onion. Cook, stirring occasionally, until onion is soft (about 7 minutes). Remove from heat and let cool; then spoon into a large bowl. Add turkey, marjoram, thyme, sage, pepper, parsley, egg whites, bread crumbs, and milk; mix lightly.

2 Pat turkey mixture into a 5- by 9-inch (12.5- by 23-cm) loaf pan. Bake in a 350°F (175°C) oven until browned on top and no longer pink in center; cut to test (about 1 hour). Drain and discard fat from pan, then invert pan and turn loaf out onto a platter. Serve loaf hot; or let cool, then cover and refrigerate for up to 1 day.

1 tablespoon butter or margarine

2 medium-size tart green-skinned apples
(about 12 oz./340 g total),
cored and chopped

1 medium-size onion (about 6 oz./170 g),
chopped

1½ pounds (680 g) ground skinless
turkey breast

1½ teaspoons dried marjoram

1 teaspoon dried thyme

1 teaspoon dried sage

1 teaspoon pepper

½ cup (30 g) chopped parsley

2 large egg whites

½ cup (50 g) fine dried bread crumbs

½ cup (120 ml) nonfat milk

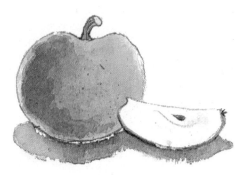

PER SERVING

EXCHANGES
½ starch, ½ fruit, 0 milk,
0 other carbohydrates/sugar, ½ vegetable,
4 very lean meat/protein, ½ fat

NUTRIENTS
237 calories (13% calories from fat), 3 g total fat,
2 g saturated fat, 76 mg cholesterol,
185 mg sodium, 19 g carbohydrates, 2 g fiber,
32 g protein, 85 mg calcium, 3 mg iron

MAKES 6 SERVINGS

Stuffed Chicken Legs with Capellini

PREPARATION TIME About 25 minutes • **COOKING TIME** About 1 hour

½ cup (20 g) cilantro leaves

½ cup (20 g) fresh basil

½ cup (40 g) freshly grated
Parmesan cheese

3 whole chicken legs (about 1½ lbs./
680 g total)

3 large red bell peppers
(about 1½ lbs./680 g total)

4 slices bacon

12 ounces (340 g) dried capellini

½ cup (120 ml) seasoned rice
vinegar (or ½ cup/120 ml distilled
white vinegar and 4 teaspoons sugar)

¼ cup (30 g) capers, drained

1 tablespoon grated lemon peel

Finely shredded lemon peel

Cilantro sprigs

Salt and pepper

While you grill the vegetables and chicken for this recipe, the capellini cooks quickly on the stovetop. You can also grill the peppers and chicken under the broiler indoors, if you prefer.

1 Combine cilantro leaves, basil, and cheese in a food processor or blender. Whirl until minced.

2 Cut a slit just through skin at joint on outside of each chicken leg. Slide your fingers between skin and meat to separate, leaving skin in place. Tuck cilantro mixture under skin, spreading evenly. Set aside.

3 Place bell peppers on a lightly greased grill 4 to 6 inches (10 to 15 cm) above a solid bed of hot coals. Grill, turning as needed, until charred all over (about 10 minutes). Transfer to a plate, cover with foil, and let cool. Pull off and discard skin, stems, and seeds. Cut peppers into strips and set aside.

4 Lay chicken on grill when coals have cooled down to medium heat and cook, turning as needed, until meat near thighbone is no longer pink; cut to test (about 40 minutes). Meanwhile, cook bacon in a wide nonstick frying pan over medium heat until crisp (about 5 minutes). Lift bacon out, drain well, and crumble; set aside. Discard all but 2 teaspoons of the drippings; set pan with drippings aside.

5 Bring 12 cups (2.8 liters) water to a boil in a 5- to 6-quart (5- to 6-liter) pan over medium-high heat. Stir in pasta and cook just until tender to bite (about 4 minutes); or cook according to package directions. Drain well and keep warm.

6 Add vinegar, capers, and grated lemon peel to pan with drippings. Bring just to a boil over medium heat. Add pasta and bacon. Cook, stirring, just until warm. Transfer to a platter. Cut chicken legs apart. Place chicken and bell peppers on platter. Garnish with shredded lemon peel and cilantro sprigs. Offer salt and pepper to add to taste.

PER SERVING

EXCHANGES
2¾ starch, 0 fruit, 0 milk,
0 other carbohydrates/sugar, 2 vegetables,
2 lean meat/protein, 1¾ fat

NUTRIENTS
457 calories (30% calories from fat), 15 g
total fat, 5 g saturated fat, 64 mg cholesterol,
858 mg sodium, 52 g carbohydrates, 2 g fiber,
28 g protein, 210 mg calcium, 4 mg iron

MAKES 6 SERVINGS

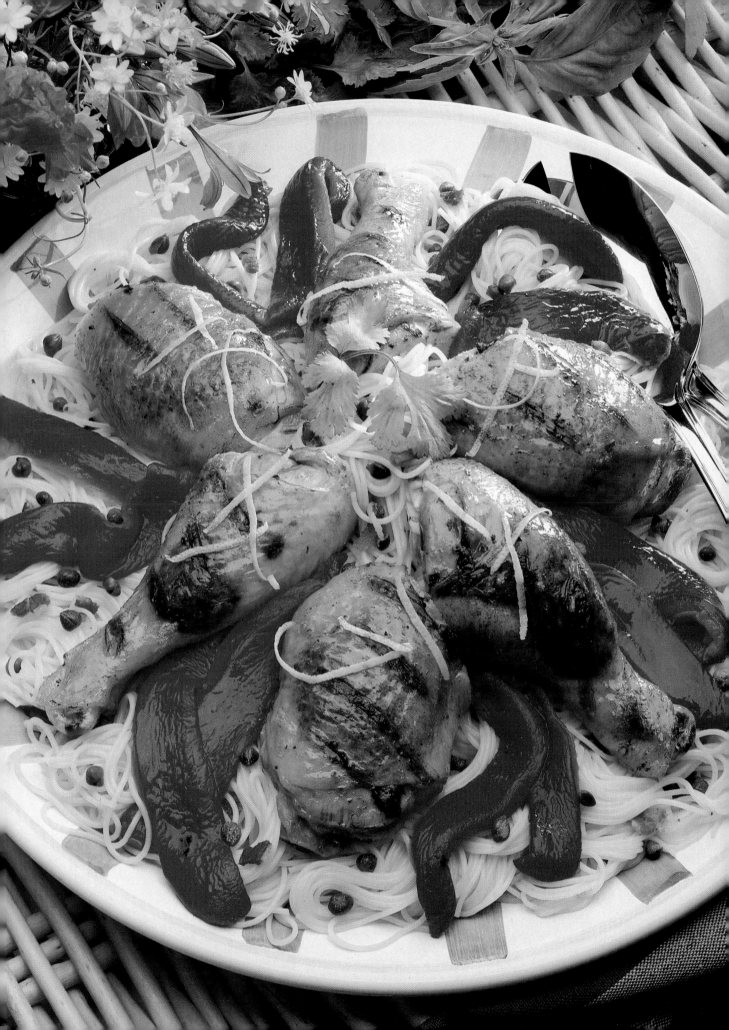

Chicken Vermicelli Carbonara

PREPARATION TIME About 25 minutes • **COOKING TIME** About 30 minutes

1 large onion (about 8 oz./230 g), finely chopped

½ teaspoon fennel seeds

1¾ cups (420 ml) fat-free reduced-sodium chicken broth

12 to 14 ounces (340 to 400 g) skinless, boneless chicken thighs, trimmed of fat and cut into ½-inch (1-cm) chunks

1 cup (60 g) finely chopped parsley

3 large egg whites

1 large egg

12 ounces to 1 pound (340 to 455 g) dried vermicelli

1½ cups (about 6 oz./170 g) finely shredded Parmesan cheese

Salt and pepper

Here's a creative low-fat version of an Italian classic. Dark-meat chicken stands in for the usual pork or bacon, and chopped onion (braised in a fennel-seasoned broth) adds a richness to the dish.

1 In a wide nonstick frying pan, combine onion, fennel seeds, and 1 cup (240 ml) of the broth. Bring to a boil over high heat; boil, stirring occasionally, until liquid evaporates and onion begins to brown (8 to 10 minutes). To deglaze, add 2 tablespoons (30 ml) water, stirring to scrape browned bits free. Then continue to cook, stirring occasionally, until onion begins to brown again. Repeat deglazing and browning steps, using 2 tablespoons (30 ml) water each time, until onions are a uniformly light golden brown color.

2 To pan, add chicken and 2 tablespoons (30 ml) more water. Cook, stirring often, until drippings begin to brown, then deglaze pan with 2 tablespoons (30 ml) water. When liquid has evaporated, add remaining ¾ cup (180 ml) broth and bring to a boil. Stir in parsley; reduce heat to very low and keep mixture warm. In a small bowl, beat egg whites and whole egg to blend; set aside.

3 In a 6- to 8-quart (6- to 8-liter) pan, cook vermicelli in 4 quarts (3.8 liters) boiling water just until tender to bite (8 to 10 minutes); or cook according to package directions. Drain well.

4 Add hot pasta to pan with chicken. Pour egg mixture over pasta and at once begin lifting with 2 forks so eggs cook and coat pasta (eggs will curdle if you delay mixing); add 1 cup (115 g) of the cheese as you mix. Pour mixture onto a deep platter and continue to mix until almost all broth is absorbed. Season to taste with salt and pepper. Offer remaining ½ cup (55 g) cheese to add to taste.

PER SERVING

EXCHANGES
3 starch, 0 fruit, 0 milk, 0 other carbohydrates/sugar, ½ vegetable, 3 lean meat/protein, ½ fat

NUTRIENTS
423 calories (25% calories from fat), 12 g total fat, 6 g saturated fat, 93 mg cholesterol, 567 mg sodium, 47 g carbohydrates, 2 g fiber, 31 g protein, 378 mg calcium, 4 mg iron

MAKES 7 SERVINGS

Chicken Capocollo

PREPARATION TIME About 15 minutes • **COOKING TIME** 10 to 12 minutes

Thin slices of spicy *capocollo* sausage enliven this quick sauté of pounded chicken breasts in a light mustard sauce. Serve the dish with thin fresh noodles or orzo (or another tiny pasta shape) and a steamed green vegetable such as broccoli or asparagus.

1 Rinse chicken and pat dry. Place each breast half between 2 sheets of plastic wrap and pound with a flat-surfaced mallet to a thickness of ⅓ to ½ inch (8 mm to 1 cm). Lay a slice of capocollo on each pounded chicken piece, pressing lightly so that chicken and sausage stick together. Set aside.

2 Heat oil in a wide frying pan over medium heat. Add onions and garlic; cook, stirring often, until vegetables are lightly browned (about 3 minutes). Then push vegetables to one side and place chicken in pan. Cook just until edges of chicken pieces begin to brown on bottom (about 4 minutes). Turn pieces over and continue to cook until meat in thickest part is no longer pink; cut to test (3 to 4 more minutes). Transfer chicken, sausage side up, to a platter; keep warm.

3 To pan, add broth, mustard, lemon juice, and basil. Bring to a boil over high heat, stirring constantly; then pour broth mixture over chicken.

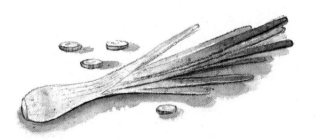

4 small skinless, boneless chicken breast halves (about 1 lb./455 g total)

4 thin slices capocollo (or coppa) sausage or prosciutto (about 1 oz./30 g total)

2 teaspoons olive oil

4 green onions (about 2 oz./55 g total), thinly sliced

2 cloves garlic, minced or pressed

¼ cup (60 ml) fat-free reduced-sodium chicken broth or dry white wine

2 tablespoons (30 ml) Dijon mustard

1 tablespoon (15 ml) lemon juice

½ teaspoon dried basil

P E R   S E R V I N G

E X C H A N G E S
0 starch, 0 fruit, 0 milk,
0 other carbohydrates/sugar, ½ vegetable,
3¾ very lean meat/protein, 1 fat

N U T R I E N T S
178 calories (26% calories from fat), 5 g total fat,
1 g saturated fat, 72 mg cholesterol,
395 mg sodium, 2 g carbohydrates, 0.4 g fiber,
29 g protein, 31 mg calcium, 1 mg iron

M A K E S   4   S E R V I N G S

Arroz con Pollo

1 can (about 14½ oz./415 g) tomatoes

About 1½ cups (360 ml) fat-free
reduced-sodium chicken broth

1 chicken (3 to 3½ lbs./1.35 to 1.6 kg),
cut up and skinned

1 teaspoon olive oil or vegetable oil

1 large onion (about 8 oz./230 g), chopped

1 small green bell pepper (about 5 oz./
140 g), seeded and chopped

2 cloves garlic, minced or pressed

1 cup (185 g) long-grain white rice

1 teaspoon dried oregano

¼ teaspoon ground cumin

¼ teaspoon pepper

1 dried bay leaf

1 package (about 10 oz./285 g) frozen
tiny peas, thawed

Salt

¼ cup (25 g) thinly sliced green onions

This classic chicken-and-rice dish is perfect for a casual Mexican-style dinner. You might complete the meal with a salad and warm corn tortillas.

1 Drain liquid from tomatoes into a glass measure. Add enough of the broth to make 2 cups (470 ml) liquid. Set drained tomatoes and broth mixture aside.

2 Rinse chicken and pat dry. Heat oil in a wide nonstick frying pan or 4- to 5-quart (3.8- to 4.8-liter) pan over medium-high heat. Add several pieces of chicken (do not crowd pan) and 2 tablespoons (30 ml) water; cook, turning as needed, until chicken is browned on all sides (about 10 minutes). Add more water, 1 tablespoon (15 ml) at a time, if pan appears dry. Repeat to brown remaining chicken, setting pieces aside as they brown. Discard all but 1 teaspoon of the drippings.

3 Add chopped onion, bell pepper, and garlic to pan; cook, stirring often, until onion is soft (about 5 minutes). Cut up tomatoes; then add tomatoes, broth mixture, rice, oregano, cumin, pepper, and bay leaf to pan. Bring to a boil.

4 Return chicken to pan. Reduce heat, cover, and simmer, adding more broth as needed to prevent sticking, until rice is tender to bite and meat near thighbone is no longer pink; cut to test (about 45 minutes). Add peas and stir until heated through. Season to taste with salt. Just before serving, garnish with green onions.

PER SERVING

EXCHANGES
2¼ starch, 0 fruit, 0 milk,
0 other carbohydrates/sugar, 2½ vegetables,
3¾ very lean meat/protein, 1¼ fat

NUTRIENTS
400 calories (15% calories from fat), 7 g total fat,
2 g saturated fat, 99 mg cholesterol,
359 mg sodium, 46 g carbohydrates, 4 g fiber,
38 g protein, 86 mg calcium, 5 mg iron

MAKES 5 SERVINGS

Oven-Fried Chicken

PREPARATION TIME About 15 minutes • **MARINATING TIME** 20 minutes • **BAKING TIME** 15 to 20 minutes

Low-fat fried chicken? Yes—if you follow our recipe. Baked in an herb-seasoned crust of cornmeal and whole wheat bread crumbs, these chicken breasts are juicy inside, crisp and crunchy outside.

1 In a shallow bowl, stir together sherry and garlic. Rinse chicken and pat dry; add to sherry mixture, turn to coat, and let stand for 20 minutes.

2 In another shallow bowl, mix bread crumbs, cornmeal, paprika, salt, pepper, thyme, basil, and rosemary. Lift chicken from marinade and drain briefly; discard marinade. Turn each chicken piece in crumb mixture to coat.

3 Lightly coat a shallow baking pan with cooking spray; arrange chicken pieces in pan. Bake in a 450°F (230°C) oven until meat in thickest part is no longer pink; cut to test (15 to 20 minutes). Serve hot or cold.

2 tablespoons (30 ml) dry sherry

2 cloves garlic, minced or pressed

4 skinless, boneless chicken breast halves (about 1½ lbs./680 g total)

½ cup (22 g) soft whole wheat bread crumbs

2 tablespoons cornmeal

1 teaspoon paprika

½ teaspoon salt

½ teaspoon pepper

½ teaspoon dried thyme

½ teaspoon dried basil

¼ teaspoon dried rosemary

Vegetable oil cooking spray

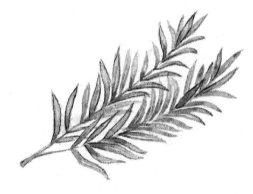

PER SERVING

EXCHANGES
½ starch, 0 fruit, 0 milk,
0 other carbohydrates/sugar, 0 vegetables,
5 very lean meat/protein, ½ fat

NUTRIENTS
231 calories (12% calories from fat), 3 g total fat,
0.6 g saturated fat, 99 mg cholesterol,
418 mg sodium, 8 g carbohydrates, 0.7 g fiber,
40 g protein, 38 mg calcium, 2 mg iron

MAKES 4 SERVINGS

Light Chicken Stroganoff

PREPARATION TIME About 45 minutes • **SOAKING TIME** About 30 minutes • **COOKING TIME** About 25 minutes

½ cup (35 g) sun-dried tomatoes, not packed in oil

1 pound (455 g) skinless, boneless chicken breasts, cut crosswise into ½-inch (1-cm) strips

Ground white pepper

1½ to 2 tablespoons all-purpose flour

1½ tablespoons (23 ml) vegetable oil

1 medium-size onion (about 6 oz./170 g), thinly sliced

8 ounces (230 g) mushrooms, sliced

½ teaspoon grated fresh ginger

½ teaspoon dried thyme

4 teaspoons cornstarch mixed with 2 tablespoons (30 ml) water

½ teaspoon sugar

1 cup (240 ml) plain low-fat yogurt

8 ounces (230 g) medium-wide eggless noodles

2 cloves garlic, minced or pressed

¼ cup (60 ml) fat-free reduced-sodium chicken broth

¾ cup (180 ml) dry white wine

2 tablespoons (30 ml) dry sherry

Chopped parsley

PER SERVING

EXCHANGES
2¾ starch, 0 fruit, 0 milk,
¾ other carbohydrates/sugar, 1½ vegetables,
4 very lean meat/protein, 1¾ fat

NUTRIENTS
526 calories (17% calories from fat), 9 g total fat,
2 g saturated fat, 69 mg cholesterol,
150 mg sodium, 62 g carbohydrates, 5 g fiber,
41 g protein, 147 mg calcium, 4 mg iron

MAKES 4 SERVINGS

To make this tempting dish, we revised a Sunset favorite containing a generous measure of butter and sour cream. The new version is far lower in fat than the original, but just as rich in flavor.

1 In a small bowl, soak tomatoes in hot water to cover until very soft (about 1 hour). Drain well, cut into strips, and set aside.

2 Sprinkle chicken with white pepper; dust with flour and shake off excess. Heat 1 tablespoon (15 ml) of the oil in a wide nonstick frying pan over medium-high heat. Add chicken, about half at a time, and cook, lifting and turning often, until lightly browned (4 to 5 minutes). Remove from pan with a slotted spoon and set aside.

3 When chicken has been cooked, heat remaining 1½ teaspoons oil in pan. Add onion, mushrooms, ginger, and thyme; cook, stirring often, until onion is soft and mushrooms are lightly browned (10 to 12 minutes).

4 Meanwhile, stir cornstarch mixture and sugar into yogurt and set aside. Also, in a 4½- to 5-quart (4.3- to 5-liter) pan, cook noodles in 2½ quarts (2.4 liters) boiling water just until tender to bite (about 10 minutes); or cook according to package directions. Drain, then arrange around edge of a warm deep platter; keep warm.

5 Stir garlic into mushroom mixture and cook for 1 minute. Then stir in broth, wine, and sherry. Bring to a boil, stirring. Add tomatoes, chicken, and yogurt mixture. Bring to a boil, stirring until sauce is thickened. Spoon chicken mixture into center of noodles and sprinkle with parsley.

Light Chicken Stroganoff ▶

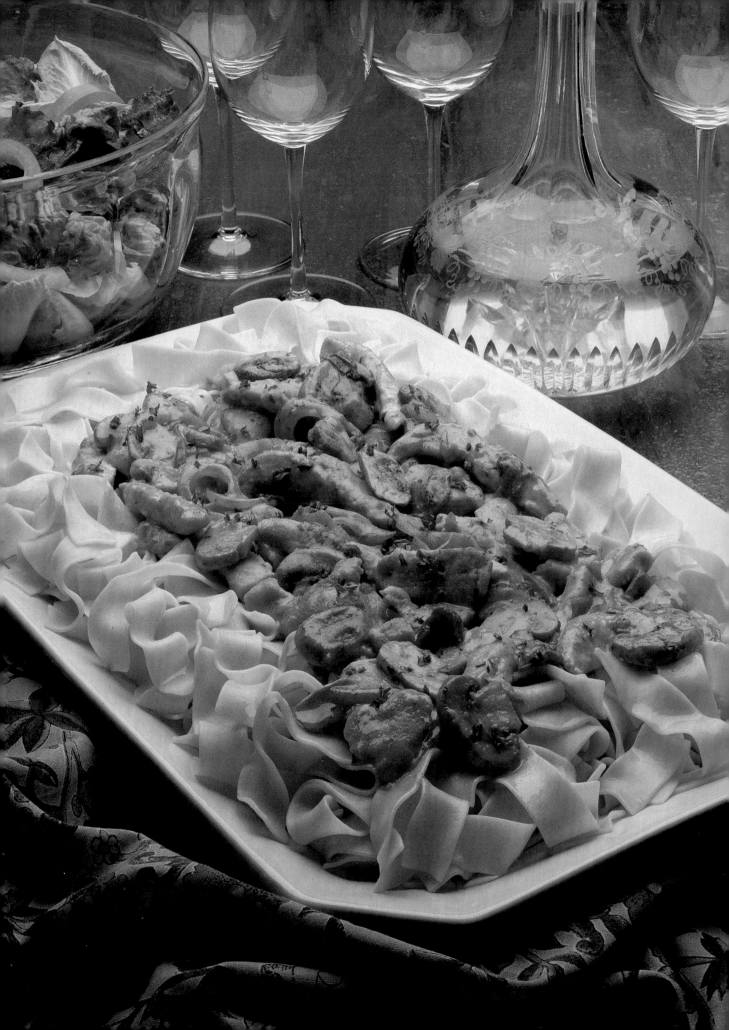

Chicken with Pumpkin Seeds

PREPARATION TIME About 10 minutes • BAKING TIME 20 to 25 minutes

4 bone-in chicken breast halves (about 1¾ lbs./795 g total), skinned and trimmed of fat

⅓ cup (30 g) roasted pumpkin seeds

1 can (about 4 oz./115 g) diced green chiles

½ cup (57 g) shredded jack cheese

Lemon or lime wedges

Crusted with a blend of pumpkin seeds, mild chiles, and jack cheese, this juicy chicken dish can be quickly prepared. At the table, add a squeeze of lemon or lime to balance the zesty seasonings.

1 Rinse chicken and pat dry; then place, skinned side up, in a 9- by 13-inch (23- by 33-cm) baking pan.

2 In a small bowl, mix pumpkin seeds, chiles, and cheese; pat evenly onto chicken.

3 Bake chicken in a 450°F (230°C) oven until meat near bone is no longer pink; cut to test (20 to 25 minutes). Serve with lemon or lime wedges.

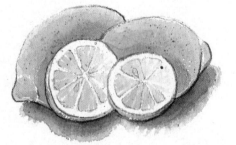

PER SERVING

EXCHANGES
¼ starch, 0 fruit, 0 milk,
0 other carbohydrates/sugar, ¼ vegetable,
4½ very lean meat/protein, 1¼ fat

NUTRIENTS
226 calories (29% calories from fat), 7 g total fat,
3 g saturated fat, 90 mg cholesterol,
334 mg sodium, 5 g carbohydrates, 0.3 g fiber,
35 g protein, 125 mg calcium, 1 mg iron

MAKES 4 SERVINGS

⁂ Seafood ⁂

Broiled Fish Dijon

PREPARATION TIME About 5 minutes ● **BROILING TIME** About 10 minutes

A bold blend of garlic and mustard complements the rich flavor of swordfish. Broiling makes this dish especially quick and easy; you can be out of the kitchen and in the dining room in under half an hour.

1 Rinse fish and pat dry. Then arrange fish and zucchini, cut side up, in a single layer on an oiled rack in a large broiler pan. Drizzle with lemon juice. Broil 4 to 6 inches (10 to 15 cm) below heat for 5 minutes. Meanwhile, in a small bowl, stir together mustard and garlic.

2 Turn fish over; spread with mustard mixture. Continue to broil until zucchini is lightly browned and fish is just opaque but still moist in thickest part; cut to test (about 5 more minutes). Sprinkle fish and zucchini with paprika and capers.

6 swordfish steaks, cut
about 1 inch/2.5 cm
thick (5 to 6 oz./140 to 170 g each)

1½ pounds (680 g) small zucchini
(about 6), cut lengthwise into halves

¼ cup (60 ml) lemon juice

2 tablespoons (30 ml) Dijon mustard

1 clove garlic, minced or pressed

Paprika

2 tablespoons drained capers

P E R   S E R V I N G

E X C H A N G E S
0 starch, 0 fruit, 0 milk,
0 other carbohydrates/sugar, ¾ vegetable,
3¾ very lean meat/protein, 1 fat

N U T R I E N T S
192 calories (28% calories from fat), 6 g total fat,
2 g saturated fat, 54 mg cholesterol,
324 mg sodium, 4 g carbohydrates, 0.6 g fiber,
29 g protein, 25 mg calcium, 2 mg iron

M A K E S   6   S E R V I N G S

Snapper Veracruz

1 teaspoon vegetable oil or olive oil

1 small green or red bell pepper (about 5 oz./140 g), seeded and chopped

1 large onion (about 8 oz./230 g), chopped

3 cloves garlic, minced or pressed (optional)

2 tablespoons (30 ml) water

1 can (about 4 oz./115 g) diced green chiles

¼ cup (32 g) sliced pimento-stuffed green olives

3 tablespoons (45 ml) lime juice

1 teaspoon ground cinnamon

¼ teaspoon ground white pepper

1 can (about 14½ oz./415 g) stewed tomatoes

4 snapper or rockfish fillets (about 8 oz./230 g each)

1 tablespoon drained capers

Named after the Mexican seacoast town where the recipe originated, snapper Veracruz features tender fillets topped with a cinnamon-spiced sauce of bell pepper, tomatoes, olives, and capers.

1 Heat oil in a wide nonstick frying pan over medium-high heat. Add bell pepper, onion, garlic, and water; cook, stirring often, until vegetables are tender-crisp to bite (3 to 5 minutes). Add chiles, olives, lime juice, cinnamon, and white pepper; cook for 1 more minute. Add tomatoes to pan and bring mixture to a boil. Boil, uncovered, stirring often, until sauce is slightly thickened (about 5 minutes).

2 Rinse fish, pat dry, and arrange in a lightly oiled 9- by 13-inch (23- by 33-cm) baking dish. Pour sauce over fish. Bake in a 350°F (175°C) oven until fish is just opaque but still moist in thickest part; cut to test (10 to 15 minutes).

3 With a slotted spoon, transfer fish and sauce to individual plates. Sprinkle with capers.

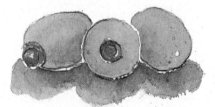

PER SERVING

EXCHANGES
0 starch, 0 fruit, 0 milk,
0 other carbohydrates/sugar, 3½ vegetables,
6 very lean meat/protein, 1 fat

NUTRIENTS
318 calories (16% calories from fat), 6 g total fat,
0.9 g saturated fat, 84 mg cholesterol,
843 mg sodium, 17 g carbohydrates, 4 g fiber,
49 g protein, 141 mg calcium, 2 mg iron

MAKES 4 SERVINGS

Curried Fish & Rice

▶◀D▶◀D▶◀D▶◀D▶◀D▶◀D▶◀D▶◀D▶◀D▶◀D▶◀D▶◀D▶◀D▶◀D▶◀D▶◀D▶◀D▶◀D▶◀D▶◀D▶◀D▶◀D▶◀D▶◀D▶◀D▶◀D▶◀D▶◀D▶◀D▶◀

PREPARATION TIME About 20 minutes   •   **COOKING TIME** About 20 minutes

A warm-and-cool fish salad is a pleasant dinner choice in any season. This one features good-tasting Chilean sea bass (richer than other sea bass). The sautéed fillets, cooked rice, and shredded lettuce are topped with a curry-seasoned sauce of tart yogurt and sweet red bell pepper.

1 Finely shred about a third of the lettuce leaves. Cover a platter with remaining whole leaves; then mound shredded lettuce on one side of platter. Set aside.

2 Heat 1 tablespoon (15 ml) of the oil in a wide nonstick frying pan over medium-high heat. Add onions and bell pepper and cook, stirring often, until pepper is soft (8 to 10 minutes). Add curry powder; cook, stirring, for 1 more minute.

3 Transfer vegetable mixture to a large bowl and stir in yogurt and water. Set 1¼ cups (300 ml) of the mixture aside. Add rice to remaining vegetable mixture and stir to combine well; then mound on shredded lettuce. Set aside.

4 Heat remaining 1 tablespoon (15 ml) oil in pan over medium-high heat. Rinse fish and pat dry. Add fish to pan and cook, turning once, until just opaque but still moist in thickest part; cut to test (8 to 10 minutes). Arrange fish on lettuce leaves; spoon reserved yogurt mixture over fish.

1 small head romaine lettuce
(about 10 oz./285 g), separated into leaves, rinsed, and crisped

2 tablespoons (30 ml) olive oil or vegetable oil

1 cup (100 g) sliced green onions

1 large red bell pepper
(about 8 oz./230 g), seeded and finely chopped

2 teaspoons curry powder

1½ cups (360 ml) plain low-fat yogurt

⅓ cup (80 ml) water

2½ cups (325 g) cooled cooked brown or white rice

4 Chilean sea bass fillets,
about 1-inch (2.5-cm) thick
(about 6 oz./170 g each)

P E R   S E R V I N G

E X C H A N G E S
1¾ starch, 0 fruit, ½ skim milk,
0 other carbohydrates/sugar, 2 vegetables,
4 very lean meat/protein, 2½ fat

N U T R I E N T S
450 calories (26% calories from fat), 13 g
total fat, 3 g saturated fat, 75 mg cholesterol,
192 mg sodium, 41 g carbohydrates, 5 g fiber,
41 g protein, 237 mg calcium, 3 mg iron

M A K E S   4   S E R V I N G S

Salmon with Asian-Style Capellini

PREPARATION TIME About 40 minutes • **COOKING TIME** About 10 minutes • **CHILLING TIME** At least 30 minutes

8 ounces (230 g) dried capellini

5 tablespoons (75 ml) seasoned rice vinegar (or 5 tablespoons/75 ml distilled white vinegar and 2 tablespoons sugar)

5 tablespoons (75 ml) lime juice

5 teaspoons (25 ml) Oriental sesame oil

¼ teaspoon ground red pepper (cayenne)

2 teaspoons reduced-sodium soy sauce

½ cup (50 g) thinly sliced green onions

5½ to 6 ounces (155 to 170 g) mixed salad greens, rinsed and crisped

1 cup (40 g) firmly packed cilantro, chopped

1 cup (40 g) firmly packed fresh basil, chopped, plus sprigs for garnish

1 large cucumber (about 12 oz./340 g), peeled, cut in half lengthwise, seeded, and thinly sliced crosswise

4 thin skinless, boneless baby salmon fillets (about 6 oz./170 g each)

Lime slices

Basil sprigs

The combination of rice vinegar, soy sauce, and Oriental sesame oil is popular in Asian cooking. In this easy-to-fix entrée, the sweet-tart flavors enhance tender pasta and crisp greens. Hot grilled salmon fillets complete the presentation.

1 Bring 8 cups (1.9 liters) water to a boil in a 4- to 5-quart (3.8- to 5-liter) pan over medium-high heat. Stir in pasta and cook just until tender to bite (about 4 minutes); or cook according to package directions. Drain, rinse with cold water, and drain well.

2 Combine 3 tablespoons (45 ml) each of the vinegar and lime juice, 4 teaspoons (20 ml) of the oil, ground red pepper, soy sauce, and onions in a large nonmetal bowl. Add pasta, lifting with 2 forks to mix. Cover and refrigerate until cool (at least 30 minutes), stirring occasionally.

3 Combine greens, cilantro, chopped basil, and remaining 2 tablespoons (30 ml) vinegar in another large nonmetal bowl. Arrange on individual plates. Top with pasta and cucumber. Set aside.

4 Stir remaining 2 tablespoons (30 ml) lime juice with remaining 1 teaspoon oil. Brush mixture over both sides of each fish fillet.

5 Place fillets on rack of a broiler pan. Broil about 4 inches (10 cm) below heat, turning once, just until opaque but still moist in thickest part; cut to test (about 4 minutes).

6 Place a hot fish fillet over pasta on each plate. Garnish with lime slices and basil sprigs.

PER SERVING

EXCHANGES
2¾ starch, 0 fruit, 0 milk,
0 other carbohydrates/sugar, 3 vegetables,
4 lean meat/protein, 1¼ fat

NUTRIENTS
570 calories (29% calories from fat), 18 g total fat, 3 g saturated fat, 94 mg cholesterol, 568 mg sodium, 57 g carbohydrates, 3 g fiber, 44 g protein, 263 mg calcium, 8 mg iron

MAKES 4 SERVINGS

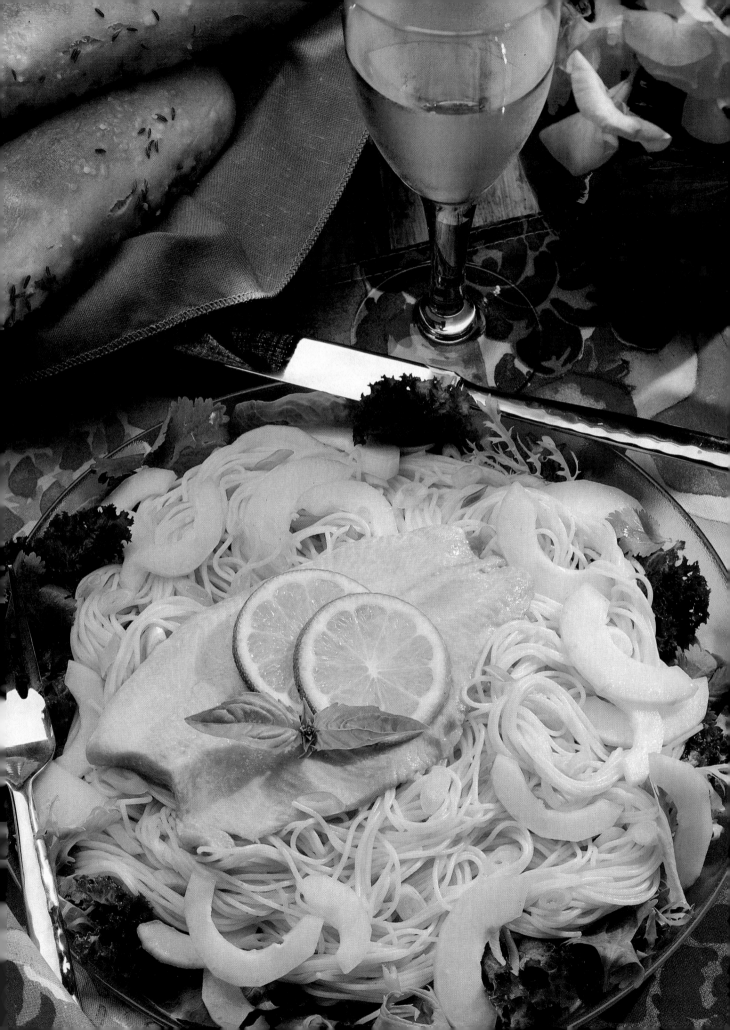

Sole Florentine

6 thin sole fillets (about 3 oz./85 g each)

2 pounds (905 g) spinach, stems removed, leaves rinsed and coarsely chopped

¼ teaspoon ground nutmeg

2 tablespoons grated lemon peel

2 tablespoons chopped parsley

¼ cup (60 ml) fat-free reduced-sodium chicken broth

¼ cup (60 ml) dry white wine

1 small dried bay leaf

4 whole black peppercorns

Filled with a lemony spinach stuffing, these delicate rolled sole fillets cook quickly in broth and white wine. If you like, you can serve them directly from the baking dish.

1 Rinse fish and pat dry. Trim each fillet to make a 3- by 8-inch (8- by 20-cm) rectangle (reserve trimmings); set aside. Finely chop trimmings; place in a bowl and add 1½ cups (300 g) of the spinach, nutmeg, lemon peel, and parsley. Stir well to combine.

2 Spread spinach mixture evenly over fillets. Gently roll up fillets and secure with wooden picks.

3 Place fish rolls, seam side down, in a 9-inch square (23-cm square) baking dish. Pour broth and wine around fish; add bay leaf and peppercorns. Cover and bake in a 400°F (205°C) oven for 10 minutes.

4 Place remaining spinach in another 9-inch square (23-cm square) baking dish. With a slotted spoon, lift fish rolls from first baking dish; arrange atop spinach (discard poaching liquid). Cover and bake until fish is just opaque but still moist in thickest part; cut to test (about 7 minutes). Remove and discard picks from fish.

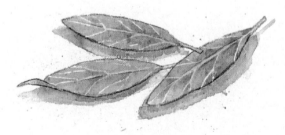

PER SERVING

EXCHANGES
0 starch, 0 fruit, 0 milk,
¼ other carbohydrates/sugar, ¼ vegetable,
2½ very lean meat/protein, ¼ fat

NUTRIENTS
108 calories (12% calories from fat), 2 g total fat,
0.3 g saturated fat, 41 mg cholesterol,
158 mg sodium, 4 g carbohydrates, 3 g fiber,
19 g protein, 130 mg calcium, 3 mg iron

MAKES 6 SERVINGS

Halibut with Tomatoes & Dill

PREPARATION TIME About 10 minutes • **BAKING TIME** About 35 minutes

Roasted cherry tomatoes, seasoned with garlic and fresh dill, make a light and colorful sauce for thick halibut fillets or steaks. If you can't find halibut, choose another firm, mild-flavored, white-fleshed fish such as rockfish, lingcod, Pacific snapper, mahi mahi, or orange roughy.

1 Arrange tomatoes, cut side up, in a 9- by 13-inch (23- by 33-cm) baking pan. In a small bowl, mix onions, garlic, chopped dill, oil, and water. Distribute onion mixture over tomatoes. Bake on top rack of a 425°F (220°C) oven for 25 minutes.

2 Rinse fish and pat dry; then cut into 4 equal pieces, if necessary. Place fish in a baking pan large enough to hold pieces in a single layer. Drizzle with lemon juice, cover, and place in oven, setting pan on bottom oven rack.

3 Continue to bake fish and tomatoes until tomatoes are lightly browned on top and fish is just opaque but still moist in thickest part; cut to test (8 to 10 minutes).

4 Transfer fish to a platter. Combine fish cooking juices with tomato mixture and stir well; spoon over fish. Garnish with dill sprigs, if desired.

1 pound/455 g (about 3 cups) cherry tomatoes, halved

½ cup (50 g) thinly sliced green onions

2 cloves garlic, minced or pressed

2 tablespoons chopped fresh dill or ½ teaspoon dried dill weed

2 teaspoons olive oil

2 tablespoons (30 ml) water

1½ pounds (680 g) halibut fillets or steaks (or rockfish or cod fillets)

2 tablespoons (30 ml) lemon juice

Dill sprigs (optional)

PER SERVING

EXCHANGES
0 starch, 0 fruit, 0 milk,
0 other carbohydrates/sugar, 1½ vegetables,
4½ very lean meat/protein, 1¼ fat

NUTRIENTS
239 calories (25% calories from fat), 7 g total fat,
0.9 g saturated fat, 55 mg cholesterol,
106 mg sodium, 7 g carbohydrates, 2 g fiber,
37 g protein, 100 mg calcium, 2 mg iron

MAKES 4 SERVINGS

Orange Roughy with Polenta

PREPARATION TIME About 10 minutes • **COOKING TIME** About 20 minutes

1 cup (138 g) polenta

4⅓ cups (1.03 liters) fat-free reduced-sodium chicken broth

½ teaspoon cumin seeds

1 large can (about 7 oz./200 g) diced green chiles

1 pound (455 g) orange roughy fillets, cut into 4 equal pieces

1 medium-size red bell pepper (6 to 7 oz./170 to 200 g), seeded and minced

1 tablespoon cilantro leaves

Salt

Lime wedges

Brighten up the dinner hour with this colorful, quick-to-fix combination. Red bell pepper and green cilantro are sprinkled over mild white fish fillets served on a bed of chile-flecked polenta.

1 Pour polenta into a 3- to 4-quart (2.8- to 3.8-liter) pan; stir in broth and cumin seeds. Bring to a boil over high heat, stirring often with a long-handled wooden spoon (mixture will spatter). Reduce heat and simmer gently, uncovered, stirring often, until polenta tastes creamy (about 20 minutes). Stir in chiles.

2 While polenta is simmering, rinse fish and pat dry; then arrange in a 9- by 13-inch (23- by 33-cm) baking pan. Bake in a 475°F (245°C) oven until fish is just opaque but still moist in thickest part; cut to test (about 6 minutes).

3 Spoon polenta onto 4 individual plates. Top each serving with a piece of fish; sprinkle with bell pepper and cilantro. Season to taste with salt; serve with lime wedges.

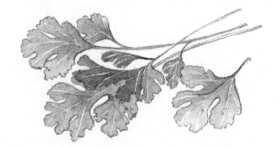

PER SERVING

EXCHANGES

2 starch, 0 fruit, 0 milk,
0 other carbohydrates/sugar, 1 vegetable,
2¼ medium-fat meat/protein, 0 fat

NUTRIENTS

320 calories (30% calories from fat), 11 g
total fat, 1 g saturated fat, 23 mg cholesterol,
501 mg sodium, 34 g carbohydrates, 3 g fiber,
24 g protein, 29 mg calcium, 2 mg iron

MAKES 4 SERVINGS

Grilled Fish Tacos

PREPARATION TIME About 30 minutes • MARINATING TIME At least 15 minutes • GRILLING TIME About 10 minutes

Lime- and tequila-marinated fish makes an unusual filling for warm tortillas. A crunchy slaw and your favorite salsa go into the tacos as well; alongside, you might serve simmered black beans.

1 Rinse fish, pat dry, and place in a wide, shallow bowl. Stir together ¼ cup (60 ml) of the lime juice and tequila (if used); pour over fish. Turn fish to coat; then cover and refrigerate for at least 15 minutes or up to 4 hours, turning occasionally.

2 Meanwhile, prepare cilantro slaw. In a large bowl, combine green and red cabbage, cilantro, remaining ¼ cup (60 ml) of the lime juice, oil, cumin seeds, and sugar. Season to taste with salt and pepper. (At this point, you may cover and refrigerate for up to 4 hours.)

3 Lift fish from marinade and drain briefly; discard any remaining marinade. Place fish on a lightly oiled grill 4 to 6 inches (10 to 15 cm) above a solid bed of medium-hot coals. Cook, turning once or twice, until fish is lightly browned on outside and just opaque but still moist in thickest part; cut to test (about 10 minutes).

4 Transfer fish to a platter. To assemble tacos, heat tortillas on grill, turning often with tongs, just until softened (15 to 20 seconds). Cut off chunks of fish (removing any bones and skin) and place in tortillas; add salsa, cilantro slaw, and sour cream to taste, if desired. Roll to enclose. Also offer slaw as a side dish.

1¾ to 2 pounds (795 to 905 g) firm-textured white-fleshed fish fillets or steaks such as Chilean sea bass, swordfish, or sturgeon (1½ to 2 inches/3.5 to 5 cm thick)

½ cup (120 ml) lime juice

3 tablespoons (45 ml) tequila (optional)

3 cups (210 g) finely shredded green cabbage

3 cups (210 g) finely shredded red cabbage

1 cup (40 g) firmly packed cilantro leaves, minced

1 tablespoon (15 ml) olive oil

½ teaspoon cumin seeds

1 teaspoon sugar

Salt and pepper

6 flour tortillas (each 7 to 9 inches/18 to 23 cm in diameter) or corn tortillas (each about 6 inches/15 cm in diameter)

About 1 cup (240 ml) purchased or homemade salsa

Reduced-fat sour cream or plain nonfat yogurt (optional)

PER SERVING

EXCHANGES

1¼ starch, 0 fruit, 0 milk, 0 other carbohydrates/sugar, 1½ vegetables, 3¼ very lean meat/protein, 1½ fat

NUTRIENTS

310 calories (23% calories from fat), 8 g total fat, 1 g saturated fat, 58 mg cholesterol, 705 mg sodium, 28 g carbohydrates, 3 g fiber, 30 g protein, 99 mg calcium, 2 mg iron

MAKES 6 SERVINGS

Shrimp with Black Bean Sauce

PREPARATION TIME About 30 minutes • **COOKING TIME** About 10 minutes

3 tablespoons fermented salted black beans, rinsed and drained

4 ounces (115 g) lean ground pork

1 large red bell pepper (about 8 oz./ 230 g), seeded and finely chopped

12 ounces (340 g) mushrooms, thinly sliced

3 cloves garlic, minced or pressed

1 tablespoon minced fresh ginger

1 cup (240 ml) fat-free reduced-sodium chicken broth

2 tablespoons (30 ml) oyster sauce

1 tablespoon cornstarch

1 tablespoon (15 ml) vegetable oil or olive oil

12 ounces (340 g) shelled, deveined medium-size raw shrimp (about 36 per lb.)

6 green onions (about 3 oz./85 g total), thinly sliced

6 cups (420 g) finely shredded napa cabbage

This quick stir-fry is sure to win the approval of time-conscious cooks and discriminating diners alike. Sweet shrimp and vegetables in a savory black bean sauce are served on a crisp bed of shredded napa cabbage. Accompany the dish with breadsticks and iced tea. Because the fermented black beans are very salty, rinse them before using.

1 In a large bowl, mix beans, pork, bell pepper, mushrooms, garlic, and ginger. In a small bowl, stir together broth, oyster sauce, and cornstarch; set aside.

2 Heat oil in a wide nonstick frying pan over high heat. Add shrimp and cook, stirring, until just opaque in center; cut to test (2 to 3 minutes). Remove from pan and set aside.

3 Add pork-mushroom mixture to pan and cook, stirring often, until meat is lightly browned (about 5 minutes). Add broth mixture and bring to a boil, stirring. Mix in shrimp and onions. Arrange cabbage on a platter and top with shrimp mixture.

PER SERVING

EXCHANGES
0 starch, 0 fruit, 0 milk,
0 other carbohydrates/sugar, 2½ vegetables,
2 very lean meat/protein, 1¼ fat

NUTRIENTS
174 calories (30% calories from fat), 6 g total fat,
1 g saturated fat, 99 mg cholesterol,
586 mg sodium, 12 g carbohydrates, 2 g fiber,
20 g protein, 119 mg calcium, 3 mg iron

MAKES 6 SERVINGS

Cajun Scallops & Brown Rice

▶◀

PREPARATION TIME About 10 minutes • **COOKING TIME** About 45 minutes

Your guests will surely be tempted by this bay scallop dish. It's spicy, but a light cream sauce helps keep the heat under control. Serve over brown rice, with a medley of seasonal vegetables on the side.

1 In a 3- to 4-quart (2.8- to 3.8-liter) pan, bring 3½ cups (830 ml) of the broth to a boil over high heat. Add rice; reduce heat, cover, and simmer until rice is tender to bite (about 45 minutes).

2 About 10 minutes before rice is done, rinse scallops and pat dry; then mix with paprika, white pepper, and allspice. Heat oil in a wide nonstick frying pan over high heat. Add scallops and cook, turning often with a wide spatula, until just opaque in center; cut to test (2 to 3 minutes). With a slotted spoon, transfer scallops to a bowl.

3 Bring pan juices to a boil over high heat; boil, uncovered, until reduced to ¼ cup (60 ml). Add remaining 1 cup (240 ml) broth and return to a boil. Stir in cornstarch mixture; bring to a boil, stirring. Stir in sour cream and scallops. Serve over rice; garnish with parsley sprigs.

4½ cups (1 liter) fat-free reduced-sodium chicken broth

1½ cups (278 g) long-grain brown rice

1½ pounds (680 g) bay scallops

1 teaspoon paprika

½ teaspoon ground white pepper

¼ teaspoon ground allspice

2 teaspoons olive oil

1½ tablespoons cornstarch blended with ⅓ cup (80 ml) cold water

½ cup (120 ml) reduced-fat sour cream

Parsley sprigs

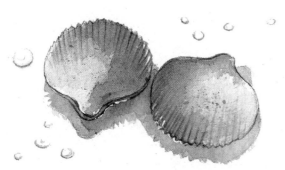

PER SERVING

EXCHANGES
2¾ starch, 0 fruit, 0 milk,
0 other carbohydrates/sugar, 0 vegetables,
2½ very lean meat/protein, 1½ fat

NUTRIENTS
346 calories (21% calories from fat), 8 g total fat,
3 g saturated fat, 44 mg cholesterol,
283 mg sodium, 43 g carbohydrates, 2 g fiber,
27 g protein, 52 mg calcium, 1 mg iron

MAKES 6 SERVINGS

Linguine with Lemon-Basil Seafood

PREPARATION TIME About 1 hour • **COOKING TIME** About 30 minutes

3 cups (710 ml) fat-free reduced-sodium chicken broth

1½ cups (360 ml) dry white wine

2 pounds (905 g) large shrimp (31 to 35 per lb.), shelled and deveined

1 pound (455 g) bay scallops, rinsed and drained

36 to 48 small mussels or small hard-shell clams in shell, suitable for steaming, scrubbed

1 tablespoon finely grated lemon peel

¾ cup (180 ml) lemon juice

¼ cup (60 ml) olive oil

3 tablespoons (45 ml) honey

1½ teaspoons coarsely ground pepper

½ cup (80 g) minced shallots

2 tablespoons chopped fresh basil or 2 teaspoons dried basil

2 or 3 cloves garlic, minced or pressed

2 pounds (905 g) dried linguine

3 tablespoons chopped parsley

Thin lemon slices

PER SERVING

EXCHANGES
4 starch, 0 fruit, 0 milk,
¼ other carbohydrates/sugar, 1½ vegetables,
3 very lean meat/protein, 1¾ fat

NUTRIENTS
518 calories (15% calories from fat), 9 g total fat,
1 g saturated fat, 124 mg cholesterol,
271 mg sodium, 71 g carbohydrates, 2 g fiber,
35 g protein, 80 mg calcium, 6 mg iron

MAKES 11 SERVINGS

This spectacular entrée of assorted shellfish is presented on a bed of linguine. Steeping the shrimp, scallops, and mussels helps to preserve their delicate flavors and textures.

1 Combine broth, wine, and 2 cups (470 ml) water in a 6- to 8-quart (6- to 8-liter) pan. Bring to a boil over high heat. Add shrimp. Cover tightly, remove from heat, and let stand just until shrimp are opaque in center; cut to test (about 3 minutes). With a slotted spoon, transfer shrimp to a large bowl; keep warm.

2 Return broth to a boil. Add scallops. Cover tightly, remove from heat, and let stand just until scallops are opaque in center; cut to test (about 3 minutes). With a slotted spoon, transfer scallops to bowl with shrimp; keep warm.

3 Return broth to a boil. Add mussels; reduce heat, cover, and boil gently until shells pop open (5 to 10 minutes). With a slotted spoon, transfer mussels to bowl with seafood; discard any unopened shells.

4 Pour broth from pan into a 2-quart (1.9-liter) measure, leaving sediment in pan. Measure 1¾ cups (420 ml) of the broth and reserve for dressing. Drain any liquid from cooked seafood into remaining broth; reserve for other uses.

5 To prepare lemon-basil dressing, in a 1- to 1½-quart (950-ml to 1.4-liter) pan, stir together lemon peel, lemon juice, reserved broth from seafood, olive oil, honey, and pepper. Bring to a boil over medium heat. Remove from heat and stir in shallots, basil, and garlic. Add 1 cup (240 ml) of the dressing to seafood and stir gently. Keep warm.

6 Bring 20 cups (5 liters) water to a boil in an 8- to 10-quart (8- to 10-liter) pan over medium-high heat. Stir in pasta, half at a time, if desired, and cook just until tender to bite (8 to 10 minutes); or cook according to package directions. Drain well and transfer to a very large platter or shallow bowl. Add remaining dressing and lift with 2 forks to mix.

7 Mound seafood over pasta, arranging mussel shells around edge of platter, if desired. Sprinkle with parsley and garnish with lemon slices.

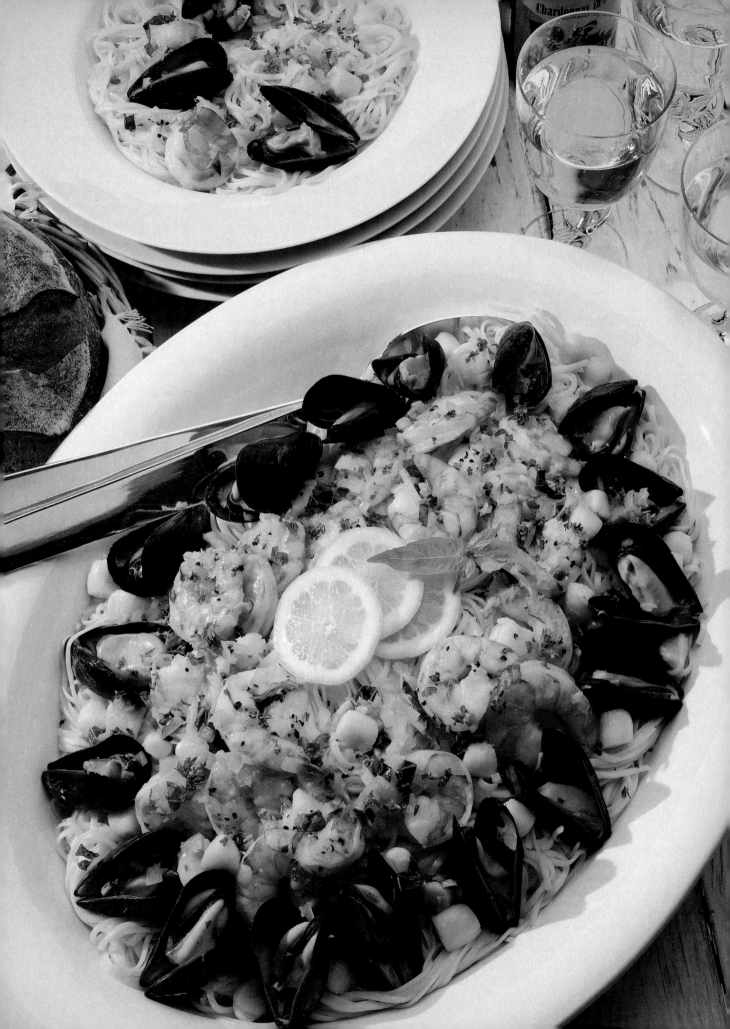

Clam Paella for Two

1 tablespoon (15 ml) olive oil

1 clove garlic, minced or pressed

¼ teaspoon ground turmeric

⅔ cup (124 g) long-grain white rice

2 tablespoons finely chopped parsley

8 ounces (230 g) cherry tomatoes, halved

⅔ cup (160 ml) dry white wine

¾ cup (180 ml) bottled clam juice or fat-free reduced-sodium chicken broth

24 small hard-shell clams in shell, scrubbed

Making traditional paella is a fairly complex undertaking, but this simplified version—starring just one kind of shellfish—is appealingly quick and easy to assemble. Serve it for supper anytime, accompanied by whole grain bread and a crisp green salad.

1 Heat oil in a wide frying pan over medium heat. Add garlic, turmeric, and rice. Cook, stirring often, until rice begins to look opaque (about 3 minutes). Stir in parsley, tomatoes, wine, and clam juice. Bring to a boil; then reduce heat, cover, and simmer for 15 minutes.

2 Arrange clams over rice. Cover and continue to cook until clams pop open and rice is tender to bite (8 to 10 more minutes). Discard any unopened clams; then spoon clams and rice into bowls.

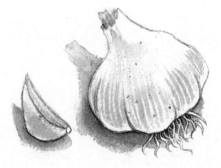

PER SERVING

EXCHANGES
3½ starch, 0 fruit, 0 milk,
0 other carbohydrates/sugar, 1 vegetable,
2½ very lean meat/protein, 2 fat

NUTRIENTS
452 calories (19% calories from fat), 9 g total fat,
1 g saturated fat, 61 mg cholesterol,
313 mg sodium, 61 g carbohydrates, 2 g fiber,
29 g protein, 133 mg calcium, 29 mg iron

MAKES 2 SERVINGS

Rice & Bean Stuffed Peppers

PREPARATION TIME About 25 minutes • **COOKING TIME** About 20 minutes • **BAKING TIME** About 45 minutes

Brown rice and black beans in a savory-sweet, raisin-dotted tomato sauce make a tasty filling for bright yellow bell peppers. Eliminate the cheese for a vegan entrée.

1 Cut off stem ends of peppers and remove seeds. If necessary, trim bases so peppers will stand upright. In a 6- to 8-quart (6- to 8-liter) pan, bring 3 to 4 quarts (2.8 to 3.8 liters) water to a boil over high heat. Add peppers; cook for 2 minutes. Using tongs, lift peppers from pan and plunge into cold water to cool; drain and set aside.

2 Heat oil in a wide nonstick frying pan over medium-high heat. Add garlic and cook, stirring, just until soft (about 2 minutes). Add 1 cup (240 ml) of the tomato sauce, wine, vinegar, cinnamon, oregano, and raisins; cook, stirring occasionally, for 15 minutes. Stir in rice, beans, and almonds.

3 Fill peppers equally with rice mixture; set upright in a shallow 1½-quart (1.4-liter) baking pan. Pour remaining tomato sauce into pan around peppers. Cover and bake in a 375°F (190°C) oven for 30 minutes. Uncover; sprinkle peppers evenly with cheese. Continue to bake until cheese is golden brown (about 15 more minutes).

6 medium-size yellow bell peppers (about 2¼ lbs./1.02 kg total)

1 tablespoon (15 ml) olive oil

2 cloves garlic, minced or pressed

1 large can (about 15 oz./425 g) tomato sauce

¼ cup (60 ml) dry white wine

2 tablespoons (30 ml) cider vinegar

1½ teaspoons ground cinnamon

1 teaspoon dried oregano

½ cup (70 g) raisins

3 cups (435 g) cooked brown rice

1 can (about 15 oz./425 g) black beans, drained and rinsed; or 2 cups (665 g) cooked black beans, drained and rinsed

¼ cup (30 g) sliced almonds

2 tablespoons grated Parmesan cheese

P E R   S E R V I N G

E X C H A N G E S
2 starch, ½ fruit, 0 milk,
0 other carbohydrates/sugar, 3 vegetables,
0 meat/protein, 1¼ fat

N U T R I E N T S
298 calories (19% calories from fat), 6 g total fat,
1 g saturated fat, 1 mg cholesterol,
585 mg sodium, 55 g carbohydrates, 8 g fiber,
9 g protein, 99 mg calcium, 3 mg iron

M A K E S   6   S E R V I N G S

Stir-Fried Broccoli, Garlic & Beans

1 package (about ½ oz./15 g) dried shiitake mushrooms

1 cup (185 g) long-grain white rice

1 medium-size head garlic (about 3 oz./85 g)

2 teaspoons salad oil

5 cups (355 g) broccoli flowerets

1 can (about 15 oz./425 g) black beans, drained and rinsed

2 tablespoons (30 ml) reduced-sodium soy sauce

1 teaspoon Oriental sesame oil

½ teaspoon honey

B roccoli, earthy-tasting black beans, and plenty of garlic distinguish this Asian-inspired stir-fry. Start the shiitake mushrooms soaking first; while they stand, you can cook the rice and do most of the other preparation.

1 Soak mushrooms in hot water to cover until soft and pliable (about 20 minutes). Rub mushrooms gently to release any grit; then lift mushrooms from water. Discard water. Squeeze mushrooms gently to remove moisture; trim and discard tough stems. Thinly slice caps, place in a small bowl, and set aside.

2 While mushrooms are soaking, in a 3- to 4-quart (2.8- to 3.8-liter) pan, bring 2 cups (470 ml) water to a boil over high heat; stir in rice. Reduce heat, cover, and simmer until liquid has been absorbed and rice is tender to bite (about 20 minutes). Transfer to a rimmed platter and keep warm. Fluff occasionally with a fork.

3 Separate garlic into cloves; then peel and thinly slice garlic cloves. Heat salad oil in a wide nonstick frying pan or wok over medium-high heat. When oil is hot, add garlic and stir-fry gently just until tinged with brown (about 2 minutes; do not scorch). Add water, 1 tablespoon (15 ml) at a time, if pan appears dry. Remove garlic from pan with a slotted spoon; place in bowl with mushrooms.

4 Add broccoli and ⅓ cup (80 ml) water to pan. Cover and cook until broccoli is almost tender-crisp to bite (about 3 minutes). Uncover and stir-fry until liquid has evaporated. Add beans and stir-fry gently until heated through. Remove pan from heat and add mushroom mixture, soy sauce, sesame oil, and honey; mix gently but thoroughly. Spoon broccoli mixture over rice.

PER SERVING

EXCHANGES

3 starch, 0 fruit, 0 milk,
0 other carbohydrates/sugar, 3½ vegetables,
0 meat/protein, 1 fat

NUTRIENTS

352 calories (12% calories from fat), 5 g total fat,
0.6 g saturated fat, 0 mg cholesterol,
516 mg sodium, 66 g carbohydrates, 10 g fiber,
15 g protein, 139 mg calcium, 5 mg iron

MAKES 4 SERVINGS

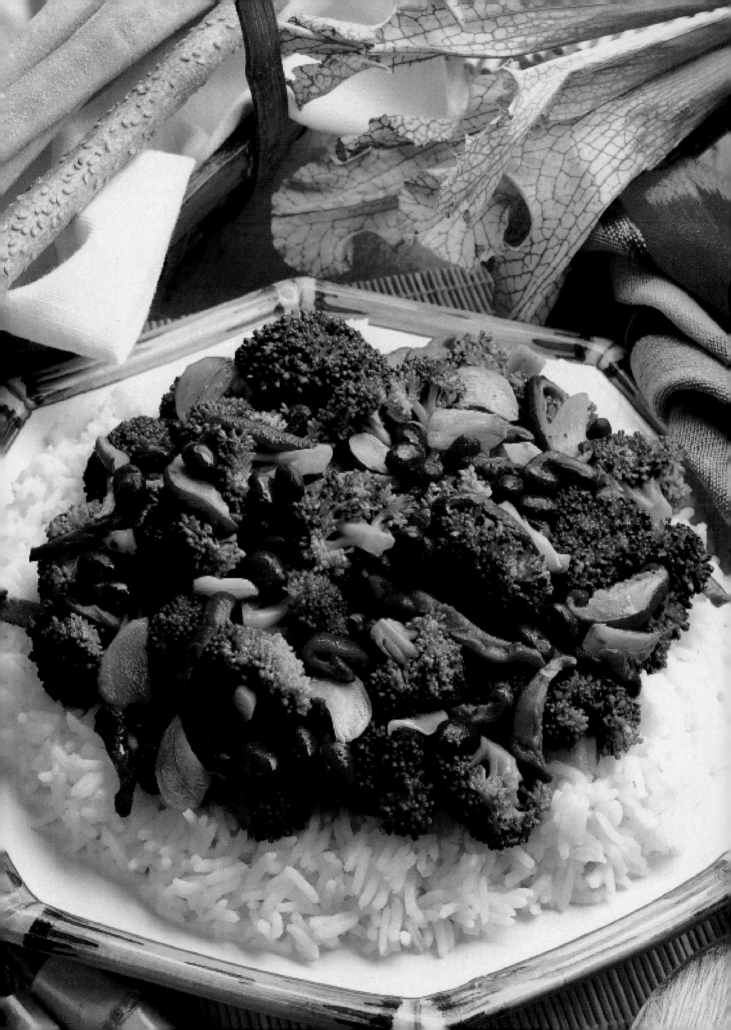

Garlic-Braised Eggplant & White Beans

PREPARATION TIME About 15 minutes • **BAKING TIME** About 20 minutes • **COOKING TIME** About 30 minutes

Olive oil cooking spray

1 small eggplant (about 12 oz./340 g), unpeeled, cut into ½-inch (1-mm) cubes

6 cloves garlic, peeled and thinly sliced

2 tablespoons (30 ml) olive oil

½ teaspoon fennel seeds

⅛ to ¼ teaspoon crushed red pepper flakes

1 teaspoon Italian herb seasoning; or ¼ teaspoon each dried basil, dried marjoram, dried oregano, and dried thyme

2 medium-size onions (about 12 oz./340 g total), thinly sliced

1 can (about 14½ oz./415 g) pear-shaped (Roma-type) tomatoes

1 can (about 15 oz./425 g) cannellini (white kidney beans), drained and rinsed; or 2 cups (370 g) cooked cannellini, drained and rinsed

8 ounces (230 g) dried medium-size pasta shells

½ cup (30 g) chopped Italian parsley

Salt and pepper

Grated Parmesan cheese (optional)

Spoon this boldly seasoned eggplant-vegetable stew over pasta shells; accompany it with a green salad and a loaf of chewy Italian bread.

1 Coat a shallow baking pan with cooking spray. Spread eggplant in pan; sprinkle with garlic, then coat with cooking spray. Bake in a 425°F (220°C) oven until golden brown (about 20 minutes).

2 Meanwhile, heat oil in a wide frying pan over medium heat. Add fennel seeds, red pepper flakes, herb seasoning, and onions; cook, stirring often, until onions are soft but not browned (6 to 8 minutes).

3 Cut up tomatoes; then add tomatoes and their liquid to onion mixture. Stir in baked eggplant. Reduce heat, cover, and simmer for 15 minutes. Stir in beans, cover, and continue to simmer until beans are heated through and flavors are blended (about 3 more minutes).

4 While eggplant mixture is simmering, in a 5- to 6-quart (5- to 6-liter) pan, cook pasta in about 3 quarts (2.8 liters) boiling water until just tender to bite (10 to 12 minutes); or cook according to package directions. Drain pasta well and divide among 5 wide, shallow individual bowls.

5 Stir parsley into eggplant mixture; season to taste with salt and pepper. Spoon equally over pasta. Offer cheese to add to taste, if desired.

PER SERVING

EXCHANGES
3 starch, 0 fruit, 0 milk,
0 other carbohydrates/sugar, 3 vegetables,
0 meat/protein, 1½ fat

NUTRIENTS
347 calories (18% calories from fat), 7 g total fat,
0.9 g saturated fat, 0 mg cholesterol,
254 mg sodium, 59 g carbohydrates, 8 g fiber,
13 g protein, 103 mg calcium, 4 mg iron

MAKES 5 SERVINGS

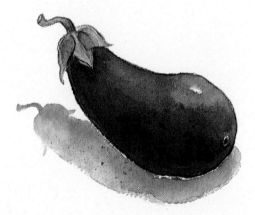

Risotto with Mushrooms

PREPARATION TIME About 15 minutes • **COOKING TIME** About 35 minutes

This simple risotto, served with bread and a crisp salad, is a lovely entrée for lunch or supper. To make it, you simmer rice and sliced mushrooms in vegetable broth until the grain is tender and creamy textured.

1 Heat oil in a wide frying pan over medium heat. Add garlic and onion; cook, stirring often, until onion is soft but not browned (about 5 minutes). Add rice; cook, stirring, until grains look opaque (about 3 minutes).

2 Stir in broth and mushrooms. Bring to a boil over high heat, stirring often. Reduce heat and simmer, uncovered, until rice is tender to bite and almost all liquid has been absorbed (about 25 minutes); stir occasionally at first, then more often as mixture thickens.

3 Remove rice from heat and stir in cheese and wine. Pour into a serving dish and garnish with parsley sprigs.

2 teaspoons olive oil

1 clove garlic, minced or pressed

1 cup (120 g) coarsely chopped onion

1 cup (200 g) short-grain white rice

2¼ cups (530 ml) canned or homemade vegetable broth

8 ounces (230 g) mushrooms, thinly sliced

¼ cup (20 g) grated Parmesan cheese

2 tablespoons (30 ml) dry white wine

Parsley sprigs

P E R   S E R V I N G

E X C H A N G E S
2 starch, 0 fruit, 0 milk,
0 other carbohydrates/sugar, 1½ vegetables,
0 meat/protein, ¾ fat

N U T R I E N T S
216 calories (17% calories from fat), 4 g total fat,
1 g saturated fat, 3 mg cholesterol,
574 mg sodium, 38 g carbohydrates, 2 g fiber,
6 g protein, 67 mg calcium, 2 mg iron

M A K E S   5   S E R V I N G S

Ratatouille-Topped Baked Potatoes

PREPARATION TIME About 25 minutes • **BAKING TIME** About 1½ hours

1 medium-size eggplant
(about 1 lb./455 g), unpeeled,
cut into ½- by 2-inch (1- by 5-cm) sticks

8 ounces (230 g) zucchini, cut into ½-inch-
thick (1-cm-thick) slices

8 ounces (230 g) crookneck squash, cut
into ½-inch-thick (1-cm-thick) slices

1½ pounds (680 g) pear-shaped (Roma-
type) tomatoes, quartered

1 large red bell pepper
(about ½ lb./230 g),
seeded and thinly sliced

1 large yellow bell pepper
(about ½ lb./230 g),
seeded and thinly sliced

1 large onion (about 8 oz./230 g), chopped

3 garlic cloves, minced or pressed

1 dried bay leaf

½ teaspoon dried thyme

½ teaspoon dried rosemary

1 tablespoon (15 ml) olive oil

6 large red thin-skinned potatoes
(about 8 oz./230 g each), scrubbed

Pepper

Fluffy baked potatoes are filled to overflowing with a variety of herb-seasoned garden vegetables—eggplant, summer squash, bell peppers, and tomatoes.

1 In a 3- to 4-quart (2.8- to 3.8-liter) baking dish, mix eggplant, zucchini, crookneck squash, tomatoes, bell peppers, onion, garlic, bay leaf, thyme, rosemary, and oil. Cover and bake in a 400°F (205°C) oven for 1 hour. Uncover and continue to bake, stirring once or twice, until eggplant is very soft when pressed and only a thin layer of liquid remains in bottom of dish (about 30 more minutes).

2 After eggplant mixture has baked for 30 minutes, pierce each unpeeled potato in several places with a fork. Place potatoes on a baking sheet; bake until tender throughout when pierced (about 1 hour).

3 To serve, make a deep cut lengthwise down center of each potato; then make a second cut across center. Grasp each potato between cuts; press firmly to split potato wide open. Spoon eggplant mixture equally into potatoes; season to taste with pepper.

PER SERVING

EXCHANGES
2½ starch, 0 fruit, 0 milk,
0 other carbohydrates/sugar, 4½ vegetables,
0 meat/protein, ½ fat

NUTRIENTS
294 calories (10% calories from fat), 3 g total fat,
0.4 g saturated fat, 0 mg cholesterol,
35 mg sodium, 61 g carbohydrates, 8 g fiber,
8 g protein, 70 mg calcium, 3 mg iron

MAKES 6 SERVINGS

Ratatouille-Topped Baked Potatoes ▶

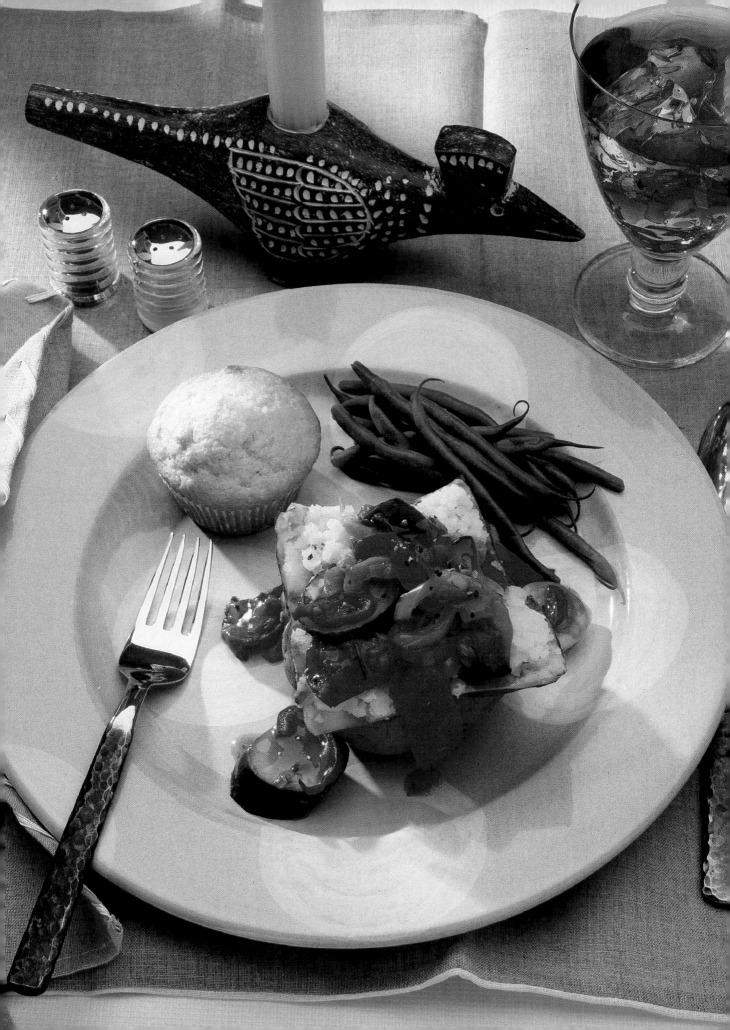

Oven-Baked Mediterranean Orzo

PREPARATION TIME About 20 minutes • **COOKING TIME** About 50 minutes

1 large can (about 28 oz./795 g) tomatoes

About 2 cups (470 ml) canned or homemade vegetable broth

1 teaspoon olive oil

1 large onion (about 8 oz./230 g), cut into very thin slivers

1 can (about 15 oz./425 g) black beans, drained and rinsed well

1 can (about 15 oz./425 g) cannellini (white kidney beans), drained and rinsed well

1 package (about 9 oz./255 g) frozen artichoke hearts, thawed and drained

½ cup (65 g) dried apricots, halved

⅓ cup (50 g) raisins

About 1 tablespoon drained capers, or to taste

4 teaspoons chopped fresh basil or 1½ teaspoons dried basil

½ teaspoon fennel seeds, crushed

1½ cups (about 10 oz./285 g) dried orzo or other rice-shaped pasta

½ cup (65 g) crumbled feta cheese

Pepper

This combination of tiny pasta, artichokes, and two kinds of beans is an easy one-dish meal. Raisins and dried apricots add their sweet flavors.

1 Break up tomatoes with a spoon and drain liquid into a 4-cup (950-ml) measure; set tomatoes aside. Add enough of the broth to tomato liquid to make 3 cups (710 ml); set aside.

2 Place oil and onion in an oval 3- to 3½-quart (2.8- to 3.3-liter) casserole, about 9 by 13 inches (23 by 33 cm) and at least 2½ inches (6 cm) deep. Bake in a 450°F (230°C) oven until onion is soft and tinged with brown (about 10 minutes). During baking, stir occasionally to loosen browned bits from casserole bottom; add water, 1 tablespoon (15 ml) at a time, if casserole appears dry.

3 Remove casserole from oven and carefully add tomatoes, broth mixture, black beans, cannellini, artichokes, apricots, raisins, capers, basil, and fennel seeds. Stir to loosen any browned bits. Return to oven and continue to bake until mixture comes to a rolling boil (about 20 minutes).

4 Remove casserole from oven and carefully stir in pasta, scraping casserole bottom to loosen any browned bits. Cover tightly, return to oven, and bake for 10 more minutes; then stir pasta mixture well, scraping casserole bottom. Cover tightly again and continue to bake until pasta is just tender to bite and almost all liquid has been absorbed (about 10 more minutes). Sprinkle with cheese, cover, and let stand for about 5 minutes before serving. Season to taste with pepper.

PER SERVING

EXCHANGES
3 starch, ½ fruit, 0 milk, 0 other carbohydrates/sugar, 2½ vegetables, 0 meat/protein, 1 fat

NUTRIENTS
358 calories (12% calories from fat), 5 g total fat, 2 g saturated fat, 9 mg cholesterol, 807 mg sodium, 66 g carbohydrates, 9 g fiber, 15 g protein, 140 mg calcium, 5 mg iron

MAKES 7 SERVINGS

Linguine with Lentils

PREPARATION TIME About 15 minutes • **COOKING TIME** About 55 minutes

Simple fare, but so satisfying! Lentils and Swiss chard, flavored in a spicy broth, combine with linguine and creamy Neufchâtel cheese for a mouth-watering entrée. Alongside, offer a plump loaf of whole grain bread.

1 In a 5- to 6-quart (5- to 6-liter) pan, bring 2 cups (470 ml) of the broth to a boil over high heat. Add lentils and cumin seeds. Reduce heat, cover, and simmer until lentils are tender to bite (about 30 minutes). Drain, if necessary; then pour into a bowl.

2 While lentils are simmering, trim and discard stem ends from chard. Rinse chard well, drain, and cut stems and leaves crosswise into ¼-inch-wide (6-mm-wide) strips (keep stems and leaves in separate piles).

3 Heat oil in lentil cooking pan over medium heat. Add chard stems, onion, garlic, and red pepper flakes. Cook, stirring often, until onion is lightly browned (about 15 minutes). Add chard leaves; cook, stirring, until limp (about 3 minutes). Add lentils and remaining 1 cup (240 ml) broth; cook just until hot (about 3 minutes).

4 Meanwhile, in another 5- to 6-quart (5- to 6-liter) pan, cook linguine in about 3 quarts (2.8 liters) boiling water until just tender to bite (8 to 10 minutes); or cook according to package directions. Drain well and pour into a warm wide bowl. Add lentil mixture and cheese; mix gently. Season to taste with salt and pepper.

---

3 cups (710 ml) canned or homemade vegetable broth

1 cup (200 g) lentils, rinsed and drained

1 teaspoon cumin seeds

1 pound (455 g) Swiss chard

2 tablespoons (30 ml) olive oil

1 large onion (about 8 oz./230 g), chopped

2 cloves garlic, minced or pressed

½ teaspoon crushed red pepper flakes

12 ounces (340 g) dried linguine

6 ounces (170 g) Neufchâtel cheese, diced

Salt and pepper

P E R   S E R V I N G

E X C H A N G E S
4 starch, 0 fruit, 0 milk,
0 other carbohydrates/sugar, 2 vegetables,
½ medium-fat meat/protein, 2 fat

N U T R I E N T S
474 calories (25% calories from fat), 13 g
total fat, 5 g saturated fat, 22 mg cholesterol,
821 mg sodium, 70 g carbohydrates, 7 g fiber,
21 g protein, 96 mg calcium, 7 mg iron

M A K E S   6   S E R V I N G S

Stuffed Shells with Red Pepper Sauce

PREPARATION TIME About 20 minutes • **COOKING TIME** About 1 hour

4 large red bell peppers (about 2 lbs./
905 g total), cut in half lengthwise

1 teaspoon olive oil

1 large onion (about 8 oz./230 g), chopped

5 cloves garlic, minced or pressed

2 tablespoons (30 ml) dry sherry,
or to taste

1 tablespoon (15 ml) white wine vinegar,
or to taste

⅛ teaspoon ground white pepper

¼ cup (20 g) freshly grated
Parmesan cheese

Salt

1 tablespoon pine nuts

20 jumbo shell-shaped pasta (about
6⅔ oz./190 g total)

1 can (about 15 oz./425 g) garbanzo beans

¼ cup (10 g) lightly packed basil leaves

2 tablespoons chopped parsley

2 tablespoons (30 ml) lemon juice

2 teaspoons Oriental sesame oil

¼ teaspoon ground cumin

Black pepper

Parsley sprigs

P E R   S E R V I N G

E X C H A N G E S
4 starch, 0 fruit, 0 milk,
0 other carbohydrates/sugar, 4 vegetables,
0 meat/protein, 1¾ fat

N U T R I E N T S
467 calories (17% calories from fat), 9 g total fat,
2 g saturated fat, 4 mg cholesterol,
424 mg sodium, 80 g carbohydrates, 8 g fiber,
17 g protein, 176 mg calcium, 5 mg iron

M A K E S   4   S E R V I N G S

Jumbo pasta shells are filled with a zesty bean mixture, then topped with a vibrant red pepper sauce. Roasted fresh peppers are lower in fat than jarred peppers packed in oil, and roasting the peppers takes only minutes.

1 To roast peppers, place peppers, cut sides down, in a 10-by 15-inch (25- by 38-cm) baking pan. Broil 4 to 6 inches (10 to 15 cm) below heat, turning as needed, until charred all over (about 8 minutes). Cover with foil and let cool in pan. Pull off and discard skins, stems, and seeds. Cut into chunks, then place in blender or food processor with any drippings. Set aside.

2 To prepare red pepper sauce, heat oil in a wide nonstick frying pan over medium-high heat. Add onion and half the garlic. Cook, stirring often, until onion is soft (about 5 minutes). Transfer onion mixture to blender with peppers. Whirl until smooth. Add sherry, vinegar, and white pepper. Whirl until desired consistency. (At this point, you may cover and refrigerate for up to 2 days; reheat before continuing.) Just before serving, add cheese. Season to taste with salt. Makes about 3 cups (710 ml).

3 Toast pine nuts in a small frying pan over medium heat, shaking pan often, until golden (about 3 minutes). Remove from pan and set aside.

4 Bring 12 cups (2.8 liters) water to a boil in a 5- to 6-quart (5- to 6-liter) pan over medium-high heat. Stir in pasta and cook just until almost tender (about 8 minutes; do not overcook). Meanwhile, drain beans, reserving liquid. Combine beans, basil, chopped parsley, lemon juice, oil, remaining garlic, and cumin in a blender or food processor. Whirl, adding reserved liquid as necessary, until smooth but thick. Season to taste with salt and black pepper.

5 Drain pasta, rinse with cold water, and drain well. Spoon half the red pepper sauce into a shallow 2- to 2½-quart (1.9-to 2.4-liter) casserole. Fill shells with bean mixture and arrange, filled sides up, in sauce. Top with remaining sauce. Cover tightly and bake in a 350°F (175°C) oven until hot (about 40 minutes). Sprinkle with pine nuts. Garnish with parsley sprigs.

Garden Patch Rigatoni

PREPARATION TIME About 20 minutes • **COOKING TIME** About 25 minutes • **BAKING TIME** About 25 minutes

This homey casserole combines plump tubular pasta and a host of vegetables in a savory Cheddar sauce enlivened with hot pepper seasoning and Dijon mustard.

1 Melt butter in a 2-quart (1.9 liter) pan over medium heat. Add celery and cook, stirring often, until soft but not browned (about 5 minutes). Add flour and cook, stirring, until bubbly. Remove from heat and gradually stir in milk; return to heat and continue to cook, stirring, until sauce comes to a boil (about 6 minutes). Add cottage cheese, Cheddar cheese, mustard, hot pepper seasoning, and nutmeg; stir until Cheddar cheese is melted. Remove from heat and set aside.

2 In a 5- to 6-quart (5- to 6-liter) pan, cook rigatoni in about 3 quarts (2.8 liters) boiling water just until almost tender to bite (10 to 12 minutes); or cook a little less than time specified in package directions. After pasta has cooked for 5 minutes, add carrots to pan; after 3 more minutes, add broccoli. Drain pasta and vegetables well; pour into a large bowl and add cheese sauce, corn, and tomatoes. Mix lightly.

3 Spread pasta mixture in an oiled 2- to 2½-quart (1.9- to 2.4-liter) casserole; sprinkle with Swiss and Parmesan cheeses. Bake in a 400°F (205°C) oven until lightly browned on top (about 25 minutes).

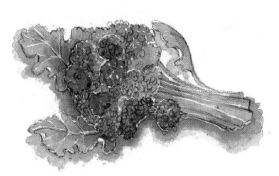

2 tablespoons butter or margarine

½ cup (60 g) thinly sliced celery

2 tablespoons all-purpose flour

2 cups (470 ml) nonfat milk

½ cup (105 g) low-fat cottage cheese

½ cup (55 g) shredded sharp
Cheddar cheese

1 tablespoon (15 ml) Dijon mustard

½ teaspoon liquid hot pepper seasoning

⅛ teaspoon ground nutmeg

8 ounces (230 g) dried rigatoni or other
bite-size tube-shaped pasta

3 medium-size carrots (about 4½ oz./
215 g total), cut into thin diagonal slices

2 cups (145 g) broccoli flowerets

1 cup (165 g) fresh yellow or white corn
kernels (from about 1 large ear corn);
or 1 cup (165 g) frozen corn kernels,
thawed

2 medium-size pear-shaped (Roma-type)
tomatoes (about 6 oz./170 g total),
seeded and chopped

½ cup (55 g) shredded reduced-fat Swiss
cheese

2 tablespoons grated Parmesan or Romano
cheese

P E R   S E R V I N G

E X C H A N G E S
2¾ starch, 0 fruit, ½ skim milk,
0 other carbohydrates/sugar, 1¾ vegetables,
1 medium-fat meat/protein, 1½ fat

N U T R I E N T S
430 calories (27% calories from fat), 13 g
total fat, 8 g saturated fat, 33 mg cholesterol,
479 mg sodium, 57 g carbohydrates, 6 g fiber,
23 g protein, 395 mg calcium, 3 mg iron

M A K E S   5   S E R V I N G S

Macaroni & Cheese

PREPARATION TIME About 15 minutes • **COOKING TIME** About 1 hour

2 slices (about 2 oz./55 g total) sourdough sandwich bread, torn into pieces

1 teaspoon olive oil

2 cloves garlic, minced or pressed

2 cups (420 g) low-fat (1%) cottage cheese

1½ cups (360 ml) nonfat milk

1 tablespoon all-purpose flour

8 ounces/230 g (about 2 cups) dried elbow macaroni

1½ cups (about 6 oz./170 g) grated sharp Cheddar cheese

⅛ teaspoon ground nutmeg

Salt and ground white pepper

Chopped parsley (optional)

This creamy, reduced-fat version of the popular casserole substitutes low-fat cottage cheese for some of the Cheddar and nonfat milk for whole milk.

1 Whirl bread in a blender or food processor until fine crumbs form. Combine crumbs, 1 tablespoon (15 ml) water, oil, and garlic in a wide nonstick frying pan. Cook over medium heat, stirring, until crumbs are crisp (8 to 10 minutes). Remove from pan and set aside.

2 Combine cottage cheese and ½ cup (120 ml) of the milk in a blender or food processor. Whirl until smooth; set aside. In a small bowl, whisk flour and ¼ cup (60 ml) more milk until smooth; set aside.

3 Bring 8 cups (1.9 liters) water to a boil in a 4- to 5-quart (3.8- to 5-liter) pan over medium-high heat. Stir in pasta and cook just until tender to bite (8 to 10 minutes); or cook according to package directions.

4 Meanwhile, heat remaining ¾ cup (180 ml) milk in another 4- to 5-quart (3.8- to 5-liter) pan over medium heat until steaming; do not boil. Add flour mixture, whisking until smooth. Cook, stirring often, until mixture begins to thicken (about 2 minutes). Remove from heat and stir in cottage cheese mixture, Cheddar cheese, and nutmeg.

5 Drain pasta well. Add to cheese mixture and mix thoroughly but gently. Season to taste with salt and white pepper. Spoon into a 2- to 2½-quart (1.9- to 2.4-liter) oval casserole. Cover tightly and bake in a 350°F (175°C) oven for 20 minutes. Uncover, sprinkle with crumbs, and continue to bake until top is lightly browned and mixture is bubbling (about 20 more minutes). Let stand for 5 minutes. Sprinkle with parsley, if desired.

PER SERVING

EXCHANGES
3½ starch, 0 fruit, ¼ skim milk,
0 other carbohydrates/sugar, 0 vegetables,
3¼ medium-fat meat/protein, ¼ fat

NUTRIENTS
554 calories (30% calories from fat), 18 g
total fat, 10 g saturated fat, 51 mg cholesterol,
861 mg sodium, 60 g carbohydrates, 2 g fiber,
37 g protein, 513 mg calcium, 3 mg iron

MAKES 4 SERVINGS

Macaroni & Cheese ▶

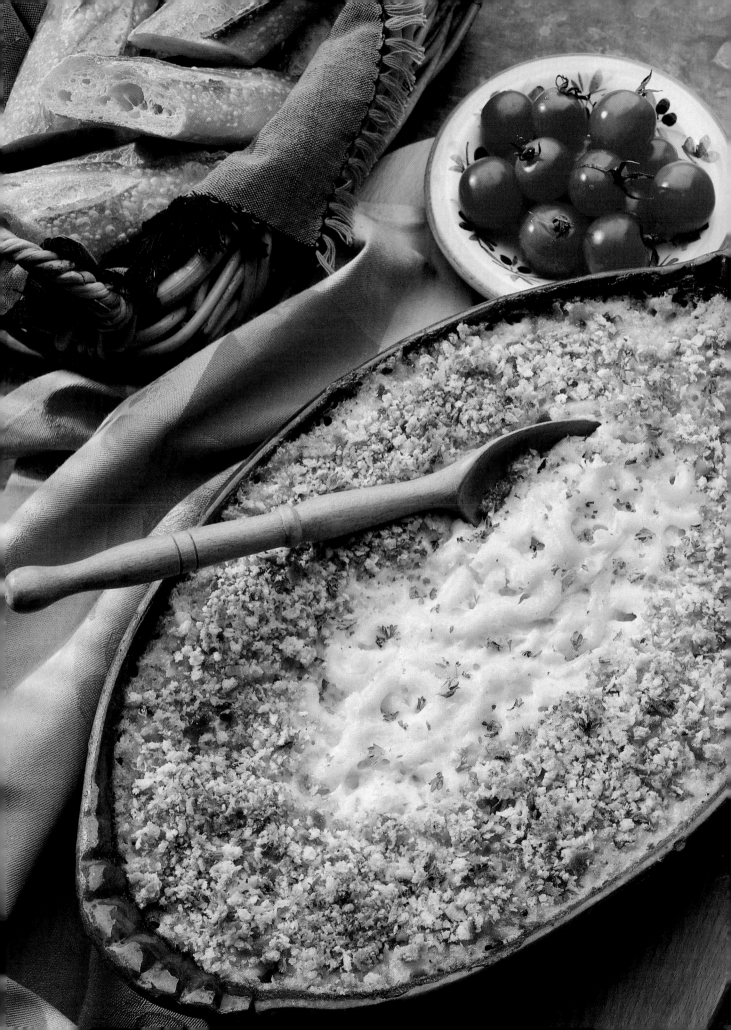

Chutney Burgers

PREPARATION TIME About 40 minutes • **COOKING TIME** About 1 hour

½ cup (113 g) mashed banana

1⅓ cups (140 g) chopped onion

⅓ cup (45 g) chopped pitted dates

⅓ cup (80 ml) pineapple juice

¼ cup (44 g) dried currants

¼ cup (60 ml) cider vinegar

3 tablespoons minced pickled ginger

½ teaspoon curry powder

2 tablespoons butter or margarine

1 teaspoon minced garlic

½ teaspoon ground cumin

½ teaspoon ground ginger

1 cup (80 g) coarsely chopped mushrooms

1 cup (185 g) coarsely chopped cooked
thin-skinned potatoes

1 cup (110 g) diced carrots
(¼-inch/6-mm cubes)

2 tablespoons chopped cilantro

⅓ cup (40 g) all-purpose flour

2 large eggs, lightly beaten

1 cup (45 g) soft whole wheat
bread crumbs

Salt and pepper

1 to 2 teaspoons vegetable oil

4 kaiser rolls, split and warmed

PER SERVING

EXCHANGES
3½ starch, 1¾ fruit, 0 milk,
0 other carbohydrates/sugar, 2 vegetables,
½ medium-fat meat/protein, 3 fat

NUTRIENTS
550 calories (27% calories from fat), 17 g
total fat, 6 g saturated fat, 122 mg cholesterol,
513 mg sodium, 89 g carbohydrates, 7 g fiber,
14 g protein, 126 mg calcium, 5 mg iron

MAKES 4 SERVINGS

These spicy all-vegetable patties are based on a mixture of potatoes, mushrooms, and carrots. Serve them in toasted rolls, accompanied by a tart-sweet chutney made from banana, ginger, and dried fruit. As an option, you might offer rinsed and crisped lettuce leaves, sliced tomatoes, sliced onion, and cilantro sprigs to add to taste.

1 To prepare chutney, in a 1- to 2-quart (950 ml- to 1.9-liter) pan, combine banana, ⅓ cup (35 g) of the onion, dates, pineapple juice, currants, vinegar, pickled ginger, and curry powder. Bring to a gentle boil over medium heat; then reduce heat and simmer, uncovered, stirring often, until chutney has the consistency of thick jam (about 30 minutes). Remove from heat; set aside to use warm or cool. (At this point, you may let cool; then cover and refrigerate for up to 3 days.)

2 Melt butter in a wide nonstick frying pan over medium heat. Add remaining 1 cup (105 g) onion and garlic; cook, stirring often, until onion is golden (about 8 minutes). Add cumin and ground ginger; stir for 1 minute. Add mushrooms, potatoes, carrots, and cilantro; cook, stirring often, until carrots are tender to bite (about 7 minutes). Add flour and cook, stirring, for 3 minutes. Remove from heat. Let cool slightly; then mix in eggs and bread crumbs. Season to taste with salt and pepper. Shape vegetable mixture into four ⅓-inch-thick (8-mm-thick) patties.

3 Heat 1 teaspoon of the oil in a clean wide nonstick frying pan over medium heat. Place patties in pan; cook until deep golden brown on bottom (4 to 5 minutes). Turn patties over; add 1 more teaspoon oil to pan, if necessary. Then cook until patties are browned on other side (2 to 3 minutes).

4 Spread rolls with chutney; serve patties in rolls.

Lean Mean Vegetable Chili

PREPARATION TIME About 20 minutes • **COOKING TIME** About 30 minutes

Because the recipe calls for canned beans, this all-vegetable chili is especially quick to prepare. If you prefer, you can make the dish with home-cooked dried beans.

1 In a 4- to 5-quart (3.8- to 5-liter) pan, combine carrots, onion, and water. Cook over high heat, stirring occasionally, until liquid evaporates and vegetables begin to brown (about 10 minutes).

2 Cut up tomatoes; then add tomatoes and their liquid, beans and their liquid, and chili powder to onion mixture. Bring to a boil; then reduce heat and simmer, uncovered, until flavors are blended (about 15 minutes).

3 To serve, ladle chili into wide bowls. Offer sour cream, if desired, and red pepper flakes to add to taste.

3 large carrots (about 10½ oz./300 g total), chopped

1 large onion (about 8 oz./230 g), coarsely chopped

½ cup (120 ml) water

1 large can (about 28 oz./795 g) tomatoes

1 can (about 15 oz./425 g) each black beans, pinto beans, and red kidney beans (or 3 cans of 1 kind); or use 6 cups (960 g) drained cooked beans plus 1 cup (240 ml) canned or homemade vegetable broth

3 tablespoons chili powder

Reduced-fat sour cream or plain low-fat yogurt (optional)

Crushed red pepper flakes

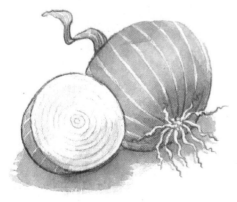

P E R   S E R V I N G

E X C H A N G E S
2 starch, 0 fruit, 0 milk,
0 other carbohydrates/sugar, 2 vegetables,
0 meat/protein, ¼ fat

N U T R I E N T S
207 calories (7% calories from fat), 2 g total fat,
0.1 g saturated fat, 0 mg cholesterol,
884 mg sodium, 40 g carbohydrates, 13 g fiber,
11 g protein, 114 mg calcium, 4 mg iron

M A K E S   7   S E R V I N G S

Black Bean Chili with Oranges

PREPARATION TIME About 40 minutes • **COOKING TIME** 2 to 2½ hours

1 pound (455 g) dried black beans

1 tablespoon (15 ml) olive oil or vegetable oil

2 large onions (about 1 lb./455 g total), chopped

2 cloves garlic, minced or pressed

8 cups (1.9 liters) canned or homemade vegetable broth

1 tablespoon coriander seeds

1 teaspoon each whole allspice

1 teaspoon dried oregano

¾ teaspoon crushed red pepper flakes

¼ teaspoon hulled cardamom seeds

4 to 6 medium-size to large oranges, mandarins, or tangelos (about 2½ lbs./1.15 kg total)

Salt

Cilantro sprigs

Reduced-fat sour cream (optional)

Fresh oranges ease the bite of this spicy meatless chili. Black beans provide protein, iron, and calcium. Serve it with corn bread or over rice.

1 Rinse and sort beans, discarding any debris. Drain beans; set aside.

2 Heat oil in a 5- to 6-quart (5- to 6-liter) pan over high heat. Add onions and garlic; cook, stirring often, until onions are tinged with brown (about 8 minutes). Stir in beans, broth, coriander seeds, allspice, oregano, red pepper flakes, and cardamom seeds. Bring to a boil; then reduce heat, cover, and simmer until beans are tender to bite (1½ to 2 hours).

3 Meanwhile, finely shred 2 teaspoons peel (colored part only) from oranges; set aside. Squeeze juice from enough oranges to make ½ cup (120 ml); set aside. Cut remaining peel and all white membrane from remaining oranges; then thinly slice fruit crosswise.

4 Uncover beans, bring to a boil over high heat, and boil until almost all liquid has evaporated (10 to 15 minutes); as mixture thickens, reduce heat and stir occasionally. Stir in 1 teaspoon of the shredded orange peel and the reserved ½ cup (120 ml) juice. Season to taste with salt.

5 To serve, ladle beans into bowls; top with orange slices. Garnish with cilantro sprigs and remaining 1 teaspoon shredded orange peel. Offer sour cream to add to taste, if desired.

PER SERVING

EXCHANGES

3¼ starch, 1 fruit, 0 milk, 0 other carbohydrates/sugar, 2 vegetables, 0 meat/protein, 1 fat

NUTRIENTS

408 calories (12% calories from fat), 5 g total fat, 0.6 g saturated fat, 0 mg cholesterol, 1,475 mg sodium, 76 g carbohydrates, 15 g fiber, 18 g protein, 184 mg calcium, 4 mg iron

MAKES 6 SERVINGS

Quick Cuke Chips

PREPARATION TIME About 20 minutes • **STANDING TIME** At least 1 hour • **CHILLING TIME** At least 1 day

Sliced cucumbers and red bell pepper strips marinated in dill-flavored vinegar are attractive and addictive—and so easy to make that the pickle jar need never be empty. Serve them with sandwiches or cold sliced meats, or include them in a low-fat antipasto assortment.

1 Cut unpeeled cucumbers crosswise into ¼-inch-thick (6-mm-thick) slices. In a large bowl, combine cucumbers, bell pepper, and onion. Add salt and dill seeds; stir well. Let stand, uncovered, for 1 to 2 hours; stir occasionally.

2 In a small bowl, combine sugar and vinegar; stir well until sugar is dissolved. Pour over vegetables and mix gently. Spoon into glass or ceramic containers, cover, and refrigerate for at least 1 day or up to 3 weeks. Drain before serving. Makes about 8 cups (1.9 liters).

3 large cucumbers (about 2 lbs./905 g total)

1 large red bell pepper (about 8 oz./230 g), seeded and cut into ½-inch (1-cm) strips

1 large onion (about 8 oz./230 g), thinly sliced

1 tablespoon salt

1 tablespoon dill seeds

¾ cup (150 g) sugar

½ cup (120 ml) white wine vinegar

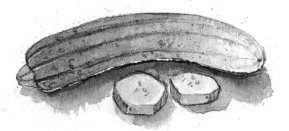

PER ½-CUP SERVING

EXCHANGES
0 starch, 0 fruit, 0 milk,
¼ other carbohydrates/sugar, 1 vegetable,
0 meat/protein, 0 fat

NUTRIENTS
36 calories (3% calories from fat), 0.1 g total fat,
0 g saturated fat, 0 mg cholesterol,
208 mg sodium, 8 g carbohydrates, 1 g fiber,
0.6 g protein, 16 mg calcium, 0.2 mg iron

MAKES 16 SERVINGS

Sherried Green Beans & Peas

1½ pounds (680 g) tender green beans, ends removed

1 package (about 10 oz./285 g) frozen tiny peas

2 teaspoons cornstarch

1 tablespoon minced fresh ginger

2 tablespoons (30 ml) reduced-sodium soy sauce

¼ cup (60 ml) dry sherry

½ cup (120 ml) water

1 tablespoon (15 ml) Oriental sesame oil

¼ cup (38 g) finely diced red bell pepper

Tender-crisp green beans and tiny peas, cooled and tossed with a simple sherry-soy sauce, make a refreshing side dish you can easily prepare in advance. Add the garnish—a sprinkling of diced bell pepper—just before serving.

1 In a 4- to 5-quart (3.8- to 5-liter) pan, cook beans, uncovered, in about 3 quarts (2.8 liters) boiling water just until tender to bite (4 to 5 minutes). Stir in peas, then drain vegetables well. Immerse in cold water until cool, then drain and pour into a wide serving bowl or onto a rimmed platter.

2 In same pan, blend cornstarch, ginger, soy sauce, sherry, and the ½ cup (120 ml) water; bring to a boil over high heat, stirring. Remove from heat and let cool; stir in oil. (At this point, you may cover and refrigerate vegetables and sherry sauce separately for up to 1 day.)

3 To serve, pour sherry sauce over vegetables; mix gently. Sprinkle with bell pepper.

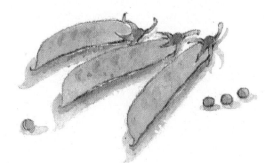

PER SERVING

EXCHANGES
¼ starch, 0 fruit, 0 milk,
0 other carbohydrates/sugar, 1¼ vegetables,
0 meat/protein, ½ fat

NUTRIENTS
71 calories (22% calories from fat), 2 g total fat,
0.2 g saturated fat, 0 mg cholesterol,
181 mg sodium, 10 g carbohydrates, 2 g fiber,
3 g protein, 32 mg calcium, 1 mg iron

MAKES 9 SERVINGS

Cauliflower with Toasted Mustard Seeds

PREPARATION TIME About 15 minutes • **COOKING TIME** About 15 minutes

Steamed just until tender, mild-tasting cauliflower makes a delicious foil for a sprightly mustard-spiked yogurt sauce. Serve this chilled side dish with juicy grilled lamb chops or a roast leg of lamb.

1 Toast mustard seeds in a small frying pan over medium heat until seeds turn gray (about 5 minutes), stirring often.

2 Place 2 tablespoons of the mustard seeds in a large bowl; stir in yogurt, minced mint, sugar, and cumin. Set aside.

3 Cut cauliflower into bite-size flowerets. Place flowerets on a rack or on a collapsible steamer in a 5- to 6-quart (5- to 6-liter) pan above 1 inch (2.5 cm) of boiling water. Cover; cook over high heat until cauliflower is tender when pierced (about 8 minutes). Immerse in cold water until cool; drain well on paper towels. Add cauliflower to yogurt-mint mixture and stir gently to coat cauliflower with sauce. (At this point, you may cover and refrigerate for up to 4 hours.)

4 To serve, arrange lettuce leaves on a platter. Spoon cauliflower mixture evenly over lettuce leaves. Sprinkle with remaining 1 tablespoon mustard seeds; garnish with mint sprigs, if desired.

3 tablespoons mustard seeds

1½ cups (360 ml) plain low-fat or nonfat yogurt

¼ cup (10 g) minced fresh mint or 2 tablespoons dried mint

2 teaspoons sugar

1 teaspoon ground cumin

1 large cauliflower (about 2 lbs./905 g), stem and leaves trimmed

1 small head romaine lettuce (8 to 10 oz./230 to 285 g), separated into leaves, rinsed, and crisped

Mint sprigs (optional)

PER SERVING

EXCHANGES
0 starch, 0 fruit, ½ skim milk,
0 other carbohydrates/sugar, 2¼ vegetables,
0 meat/protein, ¾ fat

NUTRIENTS
134 calories (26% calories from fat), 4 g total fat,
1 g saturated fat, 5 mg cholesterol,
79 mg sodium, 17 g carbohydrates, 3 g fiber,
9 g protein, 253 mg calcium, 3 mg iron

MAKES 4 SERVINGS

Almond-Zucchini Stir-Steam

½ cup (60 g) slivered almonds

2 pounds (905 g) zucchini, cut into ¼- by 2-inch (6-mm by 5-cm) sticks

2 cloves garlic, minced or pressed

2 tablespoons (30 ml) water

2 tablespoons (30 ml) reduced-sodium soy sauce

3 cups (390 g) hot cooked rice

Stir-frying is a fine low-fat cooking method—but stir-steaming in liquid is even better. These crisp zucchini sticks are cooked briefly in water and soy sauce; for a handsome presentation, spoon the zucchini over rice and top with slivered almonds.

1 Toast almonds in a wide frying pan over medium heat until golden (about 5 minutes), stirring often. Pour out of pan and set aside.

2 To pan, add zucchini, garlic, and water. Cook over high heat, turning zucchini often with a wide spatula, until zucchini is tender-crisp to bite and all liquid has evaporated (about 8 minutes). Add soy sauce and stir to combine.

3 To serve, spoon rice into a serving bowl and spoon zucchini over it; sprinkle with almonds.

PER SERVING

EXCHANGES
1¾ starch, 0 fruit, 0 milk,
0 other carbohydrates/sugar, 2 vegetables,
0 meat/protein, 1¼ fat

NUTRIENTS
224 calories (25% calories from fat), 6 g total fat,
0.7 g saturated fat, 0 mg cholesterol,
208 mg sodium, 36 g carbohydrates, 2 g fiber,
7 g protein, 67 mg calcium, 2 mg iron

MAKES 6 SERVINGS

Spiced Spinach

Here's a perfect companion for plain poached or broiled fish: vivid fresh spinach that's seasoned Indian-style, with ginger, aromatic spices, and red pepper flakes.

1 In a 5- to 6-quart (5- to 6-liter) pan, combine oil, onion, water, garlic, ginger, cumin, coriander, turmeric, and red pepper flakes. Cook over medium heat, stirring often, until onion is golden brown (about 15 minutes).

2 Add as much spinach to pan as will fit. Cook, stirring often, until spinach begins to wilt, adding remaining spinach as space permits. When all spinach has been added, increase heat to high and continue to cook, stirring, until all spinach is wilted and almost all liquid has evaporated (7 to 10 minutes). Season to taste with salt and serve with lemon wedges.

1 teaspoon olive oil

1 large onion (about 8 oz./230 g), thinly sliced

2 tablespoons (30 ml) water

2 cloves garlic, minced or pressed

1 tablespoon minced fresh ginger

½ teaspoon ground cumin

½ teaspoon ground coriander

¼ teaspoon ground turmeric

¼ teaspoon crushed red pepper flakes

2 pounds (905 g) spinach, stems removed, leaves rinsed and drained

Salt

Lemon wedges

PER SERVING

EXCHANGES
0 starch, 0 fruit, 0 milk,
0 other carbohydrates/sugar,
2¼ vegetables, 0 meat/protein, ½ fat

NUTRIENTS
73 calories (20% calories from fat), 2 g total fat,
0.2 g saturated fat, 0 mg cholesterol,
132 mg sodium, 12 g carbohydrates, 5 g fiber,
6 g protein, 179 mg calcium, 5 mg iron

MAKES 4 SERVINGS

Winter Flower Bud Rice

2 cups (200 g) cauliflower flowerets

2 cups (145 g) broccoli flowerets

1 tablespoon butter or margarine

1 large onion (about 8 oz./230 g), finely chopped

2 cloves garlic, minced or pressed

1 cup (200 g) short-grain white rice

½ cup (120 ml) dry white wine

3 to 3¼ cups (710 to 770 ml) fat-free reduced-sodium chicken broth

⅔ cup (60 g) grated Parmesan or Romano cheese

Pepper

When fresh cauliflower and broccoli are at their seasonal peak, try this savory, vegetable-studded rice as an accompaniment to your favorite veal and poultry entrées.

1 In a 3- to 4-quart (2.8- to 3.8-liter) pan, bring 2 quarts (1.9 liters) water to a boil. Add cauliflower and cook for 3 minutes; add broccoli and continue to cook until both vegetables are barely tender when pierced (about 2 more minutes). Drain, immerse in ice water until cool, and drain again.

2 Melt butter in a wide nonstick frying pan over medium heat. Add onion and garlic. Cook, stirring often, until onion begins to brown (about 5 minutes). Add rice and cook, stirring often, until rice begins to look opaque (about 3 minutes). Stir in wine and 3 cups (710 ml) of the broth; cook, stirring, until mixture comes to a boil. Reduce heat so mixture boils gently; continue to cook, uncovered, stirring occasionally, for 10 more minutes.

3 Stir cauliflower and broccoli into rice mixture. Continue to cook until rice is tender to bite and almost all broth has been absorbed (8 to 10 more minutes). Add more broth if rice becomes too dry. Stir in ⅓ cup (30 g) of the cheese; season to taste with pepper.

4 To serve, spoon rice mixture into a warm serving bowl and sprinkle with remaining ⅓ cup (30 g) cheese.

PER SERVING

EXCHANGES
1½ starch, 0 fruit, 0 milk,
¼ other carbohydrates/sugar, 2 vegetables,
½ high-fat meat/protein, ½ fat

NUTRIENTS
240 calories (24% calories from fat), 6 g total fat,
3 g saturated fat, 12 mg cholesterol,
264 mg sodium, 36 g carbohydrates, 3 g fiber,
10 g protein, 172 mg calcium, 2 mg iron

MAKES 6 SERVINGS

Winter Flower Bud Rice ▶

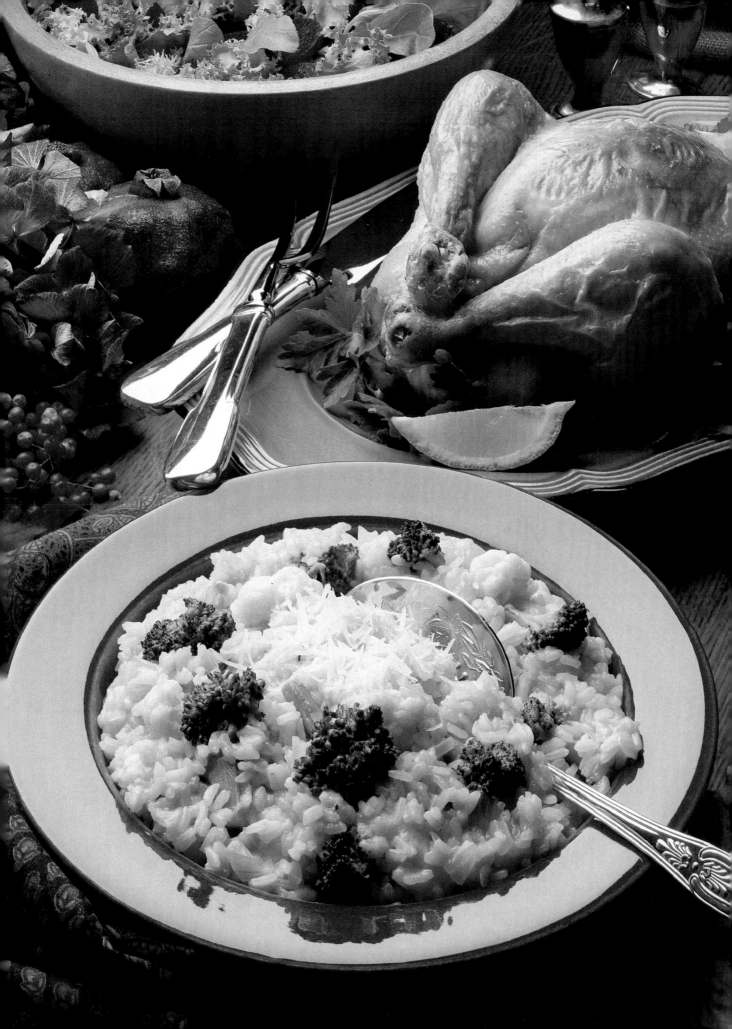

Green Rice with Pistachios

PREPARATION TIME About 25 minutes • BAKING TIME About 1 hour

2 cups (372 g) long-grain white rice

5½ cups (1.3 liters) fat-free reduced-sodium chicken broth

½ teaspoon ground nutmeg

1½ tablespoons canned green peppercorns in brine, rinsed and drained

12 ounces (340 g) spinach leaves, stems removed, leaves rinsed, drained, and finely chopped

1 cup (60 g) minced parsley

½ cup (60 g) salted roasted pistachio nuts, coarsely chopped

Choose a festive casserole like this one to partner baked turkey breast. White rice is mixed with parsley, spinach, and green peppercorns, then topped with roasted pistachios.

1 Spread rice in a shallow 3- to 3½-quart (2.8- to 3.3-liter) casserole (about 9 by 13 inches/23 by 33 cm) and bake in a 350°F (175°C) oven, stirring occasionally, until light brown (about 35 minutes).

2 In a 2-quart (1.9-liter) pan, combine 5 cups (1.2 liters) of the broth, nutmeg, and peppercorns. Bring to a boil over high heat. Stir broth mixture into toasted rice. Cover casserole tightly and continue to bake until rice is tender to bite and broth has been absorbed (about 20 more minutes); stir after 10 and 15 minutes.

3 Uncover casserole and stir in spinach, ¾ cup (45 g) of the parsley, and remaining ½ cup (120 ml) broth; bake for 5 more minutes. Stir rice mixture; sprinkle with pistachios and remaining ¼ cup (15 g) parsley.

PER SERVING

EXCHANGES
2 starch, 0 fruit, 0 milk,
0 other carbohydrates/sugar, 1½ vegetables,
0 meat/protein, 1 fat

NUTRIENTS
215 calories (21% calories from fat), 5 g total fat,
1 g saturated fat, 0 mg cholesterol,
164 mg sodium, 37 g carbohydrates, 1 g fiber,
7 g protein, 67 mg calcium, 3 mg iron

MAKES 9 SERVINGS

Oven Pumpkin Risotto

PREPARATION TIME About 10 minutes • **BAKING TIME** About 45 minutes

This creamy baked risotto owes its rich golden hue to canned pumpkin. Garnish the dish with shavings of Parmesan cheese and a grating of nutmeg.

1 In a shallow 3- to 4-quart (2.8- to 3.8-liter) casserole, combine broth, rice, pumpkin, lemon peel, and ground nutmeg. Stir to mix well. Bake in a 400°F (205°C) oven until liquid begins to be absorbed (about 20 minutes). Stir again; then continue to bake, stirring often, until rice is tender to bite and mixture is creamy (about 25 more minutes). Stir in shredded cheese.

2 To serve, transfer to a serving dish; garnish with cheese curls. If desired, sprinkle lightly with freshly grated nutmeg.

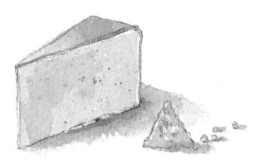

5 cups (1.2 liters) fat-free reduced-sodium chicken broth; or use canned or homemade vegetable broth

2 cups (400 g) medium- or short-grain white rice

1 can (about 1 lb./455 g) solid-pack pumpkin

1 tablespoon grated lemon peel

¼ teaspoon ground nutmeg

⅓ cup (30 g) shredded Parmesan cheese

Parmesan cheese curls, cut with a vegetable peeler (optional)

Freshly grated nutmeg (optional)

P E R   S E R V I N G

E X C H A N G E S
4 starch, 0 fruit, 0 milk,
0 other carbohydrates/sugar, 0 vegetables,
0 meat/protein, ¾ fat

N U T R I E N T S
306 calories (12% calories from fat), 4 g total fat,
2 g saturated fat, 4 mg cholesterol,
200 mg sodium, 60 g carbohydrates, 2 g fiber,
10 g protein, 115 mg calcium, 4 mg iron

M A K E S   6   S E R V I N G S

Baked New Potatoes & Apples

●━●

PREPARATION TIME About 15 minutes • **BAKING TIME** About 50 minutes

2 pounds (905 g) small thin-skinned potatoes (each 1½ to 2 inches/3.5 to 5 cm in diameter), scrubbed

2 medium-size onions, cut into 1-inch-wide (2.5-cm-wide) wedges

2 tablespoons (30 ml) olive oil

1 pound (455 g) red-skinned apples

1¼ cups (300 ml) beef broth

¾ cup (180 ml) apple juice

2 tablespoons cornstarch

¾ teaspoon ground allspice

Potatoes and apples are classic partners. Here, they bake together in a flavorful, allspice-scented sauce of beef broth and apple juice.

1 Place potatoes in a 9- by 13-inch (23- by 33-cm) baking pan. Separate onion wedges into layers and sprinkle over potatoes. Add oil and mix well. Bake in a 400°F (205°C) oven for 25 minutes, stirring occasionally.

2 Meanwhile, core apples and cut into ¾-inch-wide (2-cm-wide) wedges. Also, in a small bowl, stir together broth, apple juice, cornstarch, and allspice.

3 When potatoes have baked for 25 minutes, add apples and juice mixture to pan; stir to combine. Continue to bake, spooning juices over apples and potatoes several times, until potatoes are very tender when pierced and juices begin to form thick bubbles (about 25 minutes).

PER SERVING

EXCHANGES
1¼ starch, 1 fruit, 0 milk, 0 other carbohydrates/sugar, ½ vegetable, 0 meat/protein, ¾ fat

NUTRIENTS
191 calories (18% calories from fat), 4 g total fat, 0.6 g saturated fat, 0 mg cholesterol, 139 mg sodium, 37 g carbohydrates, 4 g fiber, 3 g protein, 15 mg calcium, 1 mg iron

MAKES 8 SERVINGS

Garlic-Roasted Potatoes & Greens

PREPARATION TIME About 25 minutes • **BAKING TIME** About 1 hour

Contrasting flavors give this hot potato salad special appeal. Potato cubes and garlic, mellowed by slow roasting, are mixed with peppery watercress and enlivened with a little red wine vinegar.

1 Coat a shallow baking pan with cooking spray. Place potatoes and garlic in pan; stir to mix, then coat with cooking spray. Bake in a 450°F (230°C) oven until well browned (about 1 hour), turning with a wide spatula every 15 minutes.

2 Drizzle vinegar and oil over potatoes. Turn potato mixture gently with spatula to loosen any browned bits. Season to taste with salt and pepper; transfer to a wide bowl.

3 Coarsely chop about half the watercress; mix lightly with potatoes. Tuck remaining watercress around potatoes. Serve hot or at room temperature.

Olive oil cooking spray

2 pounds (905 g) thin-skinned potatoes, scrubbed and cut into ¾-inch (2-cm) cubes

6 large cloves garlic, peeled and cut into quarters

3 tablespoons (45 ml) red wine vinegar

1 tablespoon (15 ml) olive oil

Salt and pepper

3 to 4 cups (140 to 180 g) lightly packed watercress sprigs, rinsed and crisped

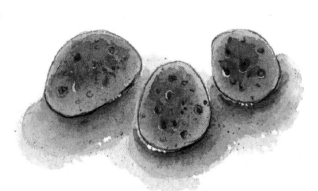

PER SERVING

EXCHANGES
2 starch, 0 fruit, 0 milk,
0 other carbohydrates/sugar, ¼ vegetable,
0 meat/protein, ½ fat

NUTRIENTS
184 calories (16% calories from fat), 3 g total fat,
0.4 g saturated fat, 0 mg cholesterol,
27 mg sodium, 35 g carbohydrates, 4 g fiber,
5 g protein, 44 mg calcium, 1 mg iron

MAKES 5 SERVINGS

Corn Custard

4 teaspoons yellow cornmeal

1 can (about 15 oz./425 g) cream-style corn

½ cup (120 ml) nonfat milk

¼ cup (60 ml) half-and-half

2 teaspoons cornstarch

¼ teaspoon salt

⅛ teaspoon ground white pepper

2 large eggs

2 large egg whites

1 package (about 10 oz./285 g) frozen corn kernels, thawed and drained

1 jar (about 2 oz./55 g) diced pimentos

Italian parsley sprigs

Despite its lush flavor and texture, this custard is surprisingly lean. To achieve velvety richness without fat, we use a combination of nonfat milk, half-and-half, and puréed cream-style corn in place of the typical butter and cream.

1 Sprinkle cornmeal over bottom of four 1¼-cup (300-ml) custard cups or ovenproof bowls, using 1 teaspoon of the cornmeal for each cup. Set cups in a large baking pan at least 2 inches (5 cm) deep.

2 In a food processor or blender, combine cream-style corn, milk, half-and-half, cornstarch, salt, pepper, eggs, and egg whites. Whirl until smooth; stir in corn kernels and pimentos. Working quickly, divide mixture evenly among cups.

3 Set pan on center rack of a 325°F (165°C) oven. Pour boiling water into pan around cups up to level of custard. Bake until custard jiggles only slightly in center when cups are gently shaken (about 1½ hours). Lift cups from pan. Let stand for 5 minutes before serving. Garnish with parsley sprigs.

PER SERVING

EXCHANGES
2½ starch, 0 fruit, 0 milk,
0 other carbohydrates/sugar, 0 vegetables,
½ medium-fat meat/protein, ½ fat

NUTRIENTS
234 calories (19% calories from fat), 5 g total fat,
2 g saturated fat, 112 mg cholesterol,
523 mg sodium, 41 g carbohydrates, 3 g fiber,
11 g protein, 75 mg calcium, 1 mg iron

MAKES 4 SERVINGS

Corn Custard ▶

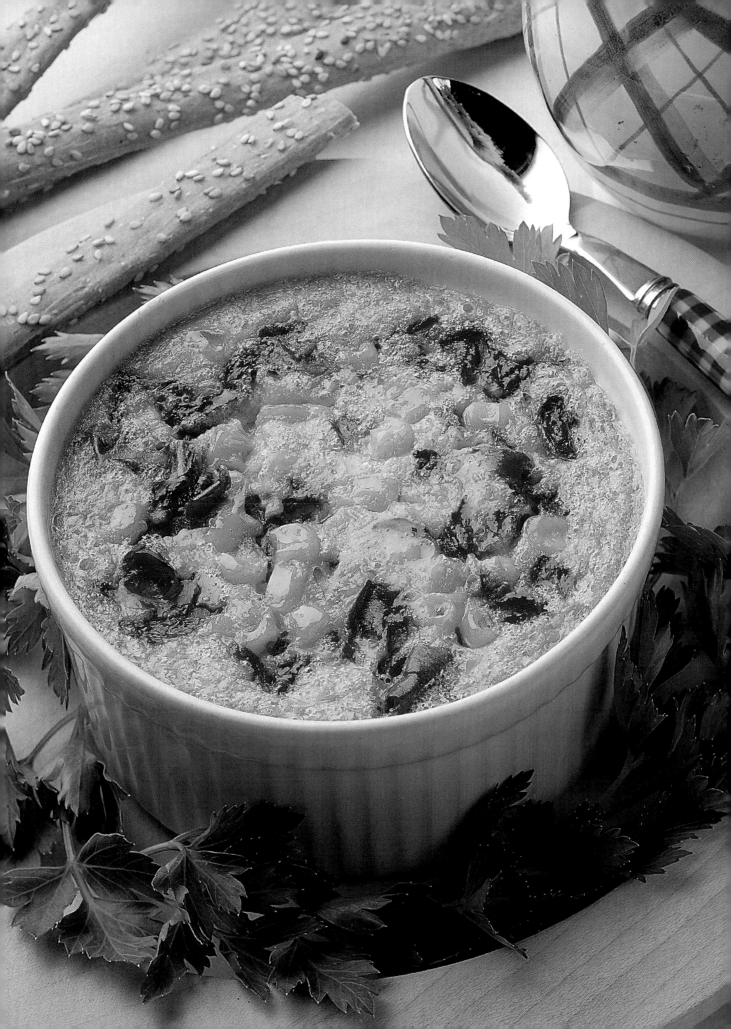

Potato & Carrot Oven Fries

PREPARATION TIME About 10 minutes • **BAKING TIME** About 45 minutes

3 or 4 large white thin-skinned potatoes (about 2 lbs./905 g total), scrubbed and cut into ½- by 4-inch (1- by 10-cm) sticks

2 pounds (905 g) carrots, cut into ½- by 4-inch (1- by 10-cm) sticks

2 tablespoons (30 ml) olive oil

Salt and pepper

Cider vinegar (optional)

Because they're baked rather than deep-fried, these crunchy potato and carrot sticks are pleasingly lean. Serve them instead of French fries with your favorite burgers.

1 In a large bowl, mix potatoes, carrots, and 1½ tablespoons (23 ml) of the oil.

2 Grease two 10- by 15-inch (25- by 38-cm) rimmed baking pans with remaining 1½ teaspoons oil and place in a 425°F (220°C) oven for 5 minutes. Then spread vegetables evenly in pans. Bake, turning once with a wide spatula, until vegetables are lightly browned and tender when pierced (about 45 minutes); switch positions of pans halfway through baking.

3 To serve, transfer vegetables to a platter or a napkin-lined basket. Season to taste with salt and pepper. Sprinkle with vinegar, if desired.

PER SERVING

EXCHANGES
2½ starch, 0 fruit, 0 milk, 0 other carbohydrates/sugar, 4 vegetables, 0 meat/protein, 1½ fat

NUTRIENTS
341 calories (20% calories from fat), 8 g total fat, 0.9 g saturated fat, 0 mg cholesterol, 97 mg sodium, 64 g carbohydrates, 11 g fiber, 7 g protein, 61 mg calcium, 3 mg iron

MAKES 4 SERVINGS

INDEX